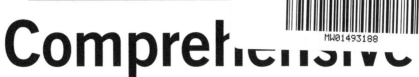

WORKB

Comprehensive

Health Skills

for High School

Fourth Edition

Publisher
The Goodheart-Willcox Company, Inc.
Tinley Park, IL
www.g-w.com

Contents

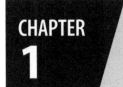

CHAPTER 1

Health and Wellness Fundamentals

Lesson 1.1   Activity A

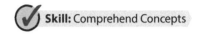
Skill: Comprehend Concepts

The Dimensions of Health

Instructions: *The three dimensions of health—physical health, mental and emotional health, and social health—are interrelated. A change in the state of one dimension often affects the other dimensions. Following each scenario, write the effects of the scenario on each dimension of the person's health.*

Scenario 1

Jermaine and his girlfriend split up. In the weeks following the breakup, Jermaine pulls away from his friends and his family. He spends hours alone in his room. He has problems sleeping through the night and often over-sleeps. As a result, he regularly skips breakfast. He has trouble concentrating in class and does poorly on his mid-term exams. To make things worse, he picks up a cold, followed by the flu.

1. Describe the effects on physical health.

   _____

   _____

2. Describe the effects on social health.

   _____

   _____

3. Describe the effects on mental and emotional health.

   _____

   _____

If Jermaine does not get help, predict how this could continue to affect each dimension of health.

4. Predict the continued effects on physical health.

   _____

   _____

5. Predict the continued effects on social health.

   _____

   _____

6. Predict the continued effects on mental and emotional health.

   _____

   _____

Scenario 2

Near the end of her senior year, Melanie is diagnosed with mononucleosis, a viral infection characterized by fatigue, sore throat, fever, and swollen lymph nodes. People with this illness can sometimes develop more serious health conditions. Melanie's doctor prescribes weeks of bed rest. Melanie cannot go to school, play sports, appear in the school play, or attend the graduation parties she was looking forward to. The doctor says it may be several months before Melanie feels normal again. After several days, Melanie feels increasingly sad and upset and falls into depression.

1. Describe the effects on physical health.

_____

_____

2. Describe the effects on social health.

_____

_____

3. Describe the effects on mental and emotional health.

_____

_____

If Melanie does not get help, predict how much each dimension of health could become more compromised.

4. Predict the continued effects on physical health.

_____

_____

5. Predict the continued effects on social health.

_____

_____

6. Predict the continued effects on mental and emotional health.

_____

_____

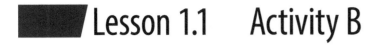 ## Lesson 1.1   Activity B

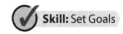 **Skill:** Set Goals

A Healthier Me

Instructions: *Reflect on your strengths and weaknesses in each area of health. Develop two or more personal goals in each area and describe steps to achieve these goals.*

Physical Health

Instructions: *Assess your current physical health.*

1. Identify your strengths: _____

2. Identify your weaknesses: _____

3. List a personal goal to improve your physical health.

   _____

4. Describe how you would go about achieving this goal.

   _____

   _____

   _____

Mental and Emotional Health

Instructions: *Assess your current mental and emotional health.*

1. Identify your strengths: _____

2. Identify your weaknesses: _____

3. List a personal goal to improve your mental and emotional health.

   _____

4. Describe how you would go about achieving this goal.

   _____

   _____

   _____

Social Health

Instructions: *Assess your current social health.*

1. Identify your strengths: _____

2. Identify your weaknesses: _____

3. List a personal goal to improve your social health.

   _____

4. Describe how you would go about achieving this goal.

   _____

   _____

   _____

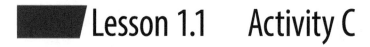 ## Lesson 1.1   Activity C

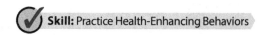 **Skill:** Practice Health-Enhancing Behaviors

Create a Quality of Life Index

Instructions: *One way to assess a person's health and wellness is to look at quality of life. This describes a person's satisfaction with various aspects of life and their ability to engage in activities of daily living. Create your own quality of life index for teens based on what areas of satisfaction you think are most important. Each area will be ranked from 1–5, with 1 meaning Very Dissatisfied and 5 meaning Very Satisfied.*

How Satisfied Are You With...

Example: the emotional support you get from your family? Ranking: 4

1. Area: _____

2. Area: _____

3. Area: _____

4. Area: _____

5. Area: _____

6. Area: _____

7. Area: _____

8. Area: _____

9. Area: _____

10. Area: _____

11. Area: _____

12. Area: _____

13. Why do you think these areas are most important for a teen's quality of life?

_____

_____

_____

_____

_____

_____

14. Do you see any obstacles that might prevent teens from feeling satisfied in these areas?

_____

_____

_____

_____

_____

_____

_____

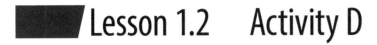 Lesson 1.2   Activity D

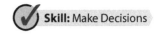

Making Healthy Decisions

Instructions: *Read the scenario about a teen whose behaviors put his health at risk. Then answer the following questions to explore a healthy decision that Sam could make to reduce his behavioral risk factors.*

> Last year, Sam felt anxious going to school because he never felt like he had friends to hang out with in the hallways or at lunch. Now, he has found a group from the track team with whom he likes spending time. Sam feels relieved that they accept him for who he is, and they can make each other laugh. Sam's friends drive him to and from school, and they vape together in the car. Sam feels like he is finally getting the hang of high school.

1. Identify the behavioral risk factor that may put Sam's health at risk, now or in the future.

   _____

2. Brainstorm and then list three specific actions Sam could take to eliminate or reduce the risk factor.

   A. Action: _____

   _____

   B. Action: _____

   _____

   C. Action: _____

   _____

3. List the pros and cons for each action you identified.

   A. Action 1: _____

   _____

   Pros: _____

   _____

   _____

   Cons: _____

   _____

   _____

   B. Action 2: _____

   _____

   Pros: _____

   _____

   _____

   Cons: _____

   _____

   _____

C. Action 3: _____

_____

Pros: _____

_____

_____

Cons: _____

_____

_____

4. Which action will most effectively reduce or eliminate Sam's risk factor? Explain your decision.

_____

_____

_____

_____

_____

_____

_____

_____

_____

_____

_____

_____

_____

_____

_____

_____

_____

_____

_____

_____

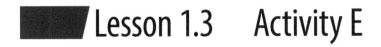 Lesson 1.3   Activity E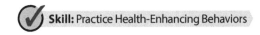

What Are the Risk Factors?

Instructions: *Risk factors can be genetic, behavioral, and environmental. They can also be either modifiable or nonmodifiable. For the following scenarios, identify and categorize the teen's risk factors. Then suggest what each teen can do to reduce or eliminate the risk factors.*

Scenario 1

Carlos is a 15-year-old who lives with his mother. When Carlos was 11 years old, he was bullied at school pretty severely. Since then, Carlos has had frequent bouts of sadness and has had problems sleeping. His father and grandmother were diagnosed with depression.

1. Identify three of Carlos' risk factors for depression. Identify whether each risk factor is behavioral, environmental, or genetic. Is each risk factor modifiable or nonmodifiable?

   _____

   _____

   _____

   _____

   _____

   _____

2. What steps can Carlos and his family take to reduce or eliminate these risk factors for depression?

   _____

   _____

Scenario 2

Arianna lives in a neighborhood where gang members hang out to sell drugs. Shootings occur on a regular basis, usually caused by gang members targeting each other; but sometimes the shootings affect bystanders. When she is 15, Arianna begins to date a 17-year-old gang member, although her parents disapprove. She often sneaks out of her home late at night to meet him in the street.

1. Identify three of Arianna's risk factors for an injury from gun violence. Identify whether each risk factor is behavioral, environmental, or genetic. Is each risk factor modifiable or nonmodifiable?

   _____

   _____

   _____

   _____

   _____

2. What steps can Arianna, her family, and members of the community take to reduce or eliminate these risk factors?

   _____

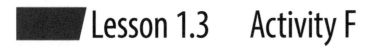 Lesson 1.3   Activity F   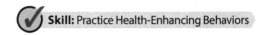 **Skill:** Practice Health-Enhancing Behaviors

Reducing Genetic Risk Factors

Instructions: *Genetic risk factors for health conditions are generally nonmodifiable. You can often make changes to your behavior and environment, however, to reduce the chance you will develop a health condition. For each of the following scenarios, identify each person's risk factors and describe what the person can do to avoid developing a health condition.*

Scenario 1

Type 2 diabetes mellitus runs in Jonelle's family. Her mother developed it when she was in her 50s. At 16 years old, Jonelle is affected by overweight. She gets very little physical activity, except for the occasional walk to school. Instead, she usually gets a ride to school. When she is not in class or doing homework, Jonelle likes to play video games with her friends. In addition, the kitchen cupboards and refrigerator in Jonelle's home are always stocked with high-calorie foods.

1. List Jonelle's genetic, behavioral, and environmental risk factors for type 2 diabetes mellitus.

_____

_____

_____

_____

2. What can she do to lower or eliminate these risk factors?

_____

_____

_____

Scenario 2

Colon cancer took the life of Josh's uncle when he was only 45 years old. Josh's uncle drank alcohol heavily, smoked cigarettes, avoided getting physical activity due to pain in his hip, and was affected by obesity. When Josh's uncle was alive, Josh hung out at his house where they played games for hours. Although he broke the law, Josh's uncle gave Josh beer and cigarettes. Josh, who is 15 years old, continues to smoke and drink, and does not get physical activity.

1. List Josh's genetic, behavioral, and environmental risk factors for colon cancer.

_____

_____

_____

_____

2. What can he do to lower or eliminate these risk factors?

_____

_____

_____

Name _____ Date _____ Period _____

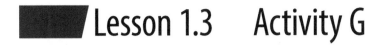 Lesson 1.3   Activity G

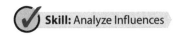

Analyzing Influences

Instructions: *Read the scenarios to examine how people's environments can affect their health. This includes physical, social, and economic environments, as well as media and technology. Then, answer the questions that follow.*

Scenario 1

> **Brooke:** Brooke lives in a safe middle-class neighborhood with walking trails, a neighborhood playground, and open fields. Brooke loves to exercise. As a young girl, she played soccer in a competitive league. Today, she continues to exercise on a daily basis. She often plays soccer with a group of neighborhood friends.
> **Charlotte:** Charlotte lives in a low-income, high-crime neighborhood. Due to her parents' financial situation, Charlotte did not play youth sports as a child. Charlotte is still cautious about going out to exercise or play with friends in her neighborhood.

1. How do Brooke's and Charlotte's environments influence their health in different ways? What specific parts of their environments are affecting their health?

_____

_____

_____

_____

_____

_____

2. What aspects of health are being affected? Describe the effects for each teen.

_____

_____

_____

_____

3. Given the situation Charlotte is in, what can she do to get more physical activity? How could exercising with a friend benefit her?

_____

_____

_____

_____

4. How can physical activity positively affect Charlotte's health?

_____

_____

_____

_____

_____

Scenario 2

Liam: Liam is raised by a supportive and loving grandmother. Growing up, his grandmother always told him to choose his friends wisely. She encouraged Liam to find friends who were happy, were smart, and followed the rules. Liam found a good group of friends, feels good about himself, and is happy.

Juan: Juan has been feeling stressed and down lately. His parents have been going through a divorce the last six months, and Juan has many unanswered questions and feels invisible in his home. His friends have been unreliable and lately have been engaging in risky behaviors such as vaping and stealing, which is creating more stress for him.

1. How do Liam's and Juan's environments influence their health in different ways? What specific parts of their environments are affecting their health?

_____

_____

_____

_____

_____

2. What aspects of health are being affected? Describe the effects for each teen.

_____

_____

_____

_____

3. What can Juan do to improve his health, given his environment?

_____

_____

_____

_____

4. How can supportive friends and family positively affect Juan's health?

_____

_____

_____

_____

_____

_____

_____

_____

Chapter 1 Activity H

Practice Test

Completion

Instructions: *Write the term that completes the statement in the space provided.*

1. The process of identifying one's state of health and taking steps to improve it is called _____.

   _____

2. While life expectancy measures the length of time a person is expected to live, the actual number of years a person lives is called _____.

   _____

3. Risk factors increase the chances a person will develop a disease or experience an injury, while _____ factors reduce these chances.

   _____

4. Health conditions that develop due to a person's genes without any other risk factors are called _____.

   _____

5. Your social environment includes your _____, or the beliefs, values, customs, and arts of a group of people.

   _____

True/False

Instructions: *Indicate whether each statement below is true or false.*

6. _____ *True or false?* A problem in one dimension of health will *not* affect other dimensions of health.

7. _____ *True or false?* Quality of life gauges a person's satisfaction with life, not just how long the person lives.

8. _____ *True or false?* Your actions can affect your health.

Multiple Choice

Instructions: *Select the letter that corresponds to the correct answer.*

9. _____ How people express their thoughts, emotions, moods, feelings about themselves, and views about the world is _____ health.
   A. physical
   B. mental
   C. emotional
   D. social

10. _____ Illness and premature death lie at one end of the health continuum, and _____ health lies at the other.
   A. perfect
   B. optimal
   C. moderate
   D. quality

11. _____ Which type of risk factor is typically nonmodifiable?
   A. genetic risk factors
   B. behavioral risk factors
   C. environmental risk factors
   D. All of the above.

12. _____ Lack of _____ due to blue light from digital devices reduces resistance to disease and impairs motor skills.
   A. sleep
   B. physical activity
   C. nutrition
   D. B and C.

13. _____ Which of the following is *not* an environmental risk factor?
   A. climate
   B. work conditions
   C. behavior
   D. geography

Matching

Instructions: *Match each key term to its definition (14–19).*

14. _____ extent to which a person experiences a healthy, happy, and fulfilling life

15. _____ choices and behaviors that affect a person's chance of developing a disease, unhealthy condition, or injury

16. _____ actual number of years a person lives

17. _____ length of time a person is expected to live

18. _____ aspects of people's lives that increase the chances they will develop a disease or disorder or experience an injury or decline in health

19. _____ presence of waste in the environment

A. behavioral factors
B. life expectancy
C. life span
D. pollution
E. quality of life
F. risk factors

Analyzing Data

Instructions: *The following chart presents the current life expectancy at birth for various countries according to the Central Intelligence Agency. Each country is listed with its ranking compared to other countries in the world. Use the information provided to answer the following questions.*

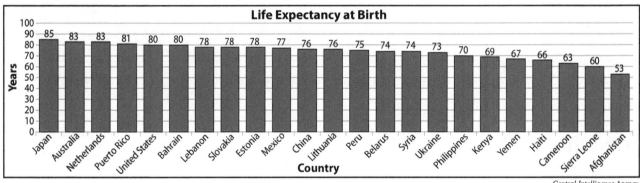

Central Intelligence Agency

Figure 1. Life expectancy at birth by country

20. What is the life expectancy at birth for people in the United States?

_____

21. How does the life expectancy at birth for people in Japan compare to that of people in Haiti?

_____

22. What are some factors that affect a country's life expectancy? Do additional research if necessary.

_____

Short Answer

Instructions: *Answer the following questions using what you have learned in this chapter.*

23. Contrast modifiable risk factors and nonmodifiable risk factors. Give two examples of each.

_____

_____

_____

_____

24. Explain why life expectancy and life span can be different due to behavioral risk factors.

_____

_____

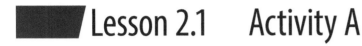

CHAPTER 2 **Health and Wellness Skills**

Lesson 2.1   Activity A

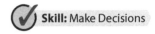

Skill: Make Decisions

Decision-Making 101

Instructions: *Identify a health or wellness problem you are currently facing. Use the DECIDE model of decision-making to guide you in finding a solution and in putting the solution into action this week.*

Step 1: Define the problem.

1. In the space below, briefly but accurately describe the problem you are facing.

   _____

   _____

   _____

Step 2: Explore alternatives.

2. List three possible solutions to the problem. Your possible solutions should contain steps or actions that you can realistically begin to take this week.

   A. Solution: _____

   _____

   B. Solution: _____

   _____

   C. Solution: _____

   _____

Step 3: Consider the consequences of each alternative.

3. List the pros and cons of each alternative you selected in Step 2.

   A. Solution 1: _____

   _____

   Pros: _____

   _____

   _____

   Cons: _____

   _____

   _____

B. Solution 2: _____

_____

Pros: _____

_____

_____

Cons: _____

_____

_____

C. Solution 3: _____

_____

Pros: _____

_____

_____

Cons: _____

_____

_____

Step 4: Identify the best alternative.

4. Identify the best alternative. Which solution best solves your problem? Why?

_____

_____

_____

Step 5: Decide on an alternative and act.

5. Describe how you will act on your chosen alternative, and then take action. Afterward, explain how you acted on your decision and what happened or will happen as a result.

_____

_____

_____

Step 6: Evaluate your decision and revise, if necessary.

6. Based on the consequences of your actions, do you think you made a good decision? Explain. If you do not think you made a good decision, which alternative do you think would work better in the future?

_____

_____

_____

Name _____ Date _____ Period _____

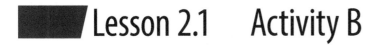 Lesson 2.1   Activity B

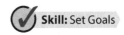

SMART Goal Setting 101

Instructions: *Record a SMART goal for improving your health and list specific steps you can take to reach that goal. An example of a SMART goal would be "I will run outside for 30 minutes every night this week." Then, each day this week, track the steps you took toward completing your goal. At the end of the week, analyze the results of your efforts by answering the questions below.*

SMART Goal for Better Health

1. Record a SMART goal.

   _____

2. List specific steps.

   A. Step 1: _____

   B. Step 2: _____

   C. Step 3: _____

   D. Step 4: _____

   E. Step 5: _____

Instructions: *Track your progress by creating a table like the one shown.*

Steps	Sun	Mon	Tues	Wed	Thurs	Fri	Sat
Step 1	X	X	X	X	X	X	X

Figure 1. Example table for tracking progress

3. What circumstances, people, or resources were helpful as you tried to achieve your goal?

   _____

   _____

4. What circumstances, people, or resources hindered your progress or became obstacles to the achievement of your goal?

   _____

   _____

5. Are you satisfied with the results of your efforts this week? Explain your answer.

   _____

   _____

   _____

6. Do you need to revise your goal or the steps you will take to reach it? If so, explain how.

   _____

   _____

   _____

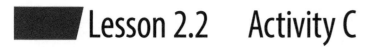 **Lesson 2.2   Activity C**

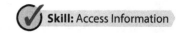

Finding Reliable Health Information

Instructions: *Find three sources of reliable information for each topic listed below. For each source, write the name of the organization and the title of the article or website page. Do not use the same source twice.*

Topic: Alcohol Poisoning

1. Website #1 (name of organization): _____

   A. Title of article or website page: _____

2. Website #2 (name of organization): _____

   A. Title of article or website page: _____

3. Website #3 (name of organization): _____

   A. Title of article or website page: _____

Topic: Acne

4. Website #1 (name of organization): _____

   A. Title of article or website page: _____

5. Website #2 (name of organization): _____

   A. Title of article or website page: _____

6. Website #3 (name of organization): _____

   A. Title of article or website page: _____

Questions

Instructions: *After compiling the above information about your sources, answer the following questions.*

1. Reflect on one of the topics. Of the sources you chose for that topic, which source was most reliable? How do you know?

_____

_____

_____

_____

_____

_____

2. Which source provided the most interesting information?

_____

3. Write three facts you learned about that topic.

_____

_____

_____

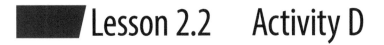 Lesson 2.2   Activity D

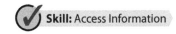 **Skill:** Access Information

Evaluating Health Information

Instructions: *Follow the instructions for each part of this activity.*

Part 1: Health Product

Instructions: *Think of a health product that you have seen advertised recently, such as a dietary supplement, essential oil, or safety equipment for a sport. Answer the following questions about this product. Do additional research if necessary.*

1. What health product did you choose? What does this product supposedly do?

   _____

   _____

   _____

2. What claims does this product or company make about its impact on health?

   _____

   _____

   _____

3. Where was this product advertised? Who do you think is the target audience?

   _____

   _____

4. Where can people buy this product?

   _____

   _____

5. How much does this product cost?

   _____

6. Are there restrictions for purchase of this product (on age, for example)? Explain.

   _____

   _____

   _____

Part 2: Research

Instructions: *Find an article that provides information about the health benefits of this product. Answer the following questions to evaluate the reliability of this information.*

1. Provide a citation for the resource you found for your health product. Include the article title, author, information sponsor, and publication date.

   _____

   _____

   _____

2. Use the following checklist to evaluate the validity and reliability of your resource.

   A. _____ Information is current up to one year.

   B. _____ Information is supported by other reliable resources.

   C. _____ Information is based on scientific research.

   D. _____ There is adequate information about the topic.

   E. _____ Facts are cited or referenced.

   F. _____ Information is reasonable (not too good to be true).

   G. _____ Information is applicable to my life stage and situation.

   H. _____ Purpose of resource is stated.

   I. _____ Resource is not making money from the information (not an advertisement).

   J. _____ Author's name is listed.

   K. _____ Author's background is trustworthy and dependable.

   L. _____ Author presents unbiased information.

   M._____ Resource is sponsored by a credible institution or organization.

   N. _____ Website address of resource ends in .gov, .edu, or .org.

3. Identify one example from your article of the author's use of science or pseudoscience for health claims. Describe this example here.

   _____

   _____

   _____

   _____

   _____

   _____

   _____

   _____

   _____

   _____

   _____

   _____

   _____

4. After your evaluation, do you think your article is a reliable source of information? Explain.

   _____

   _____

   _____

   _____

5. Would you recommend other people use this health product? Why or why not?

   _____

   _____

   _____

   _____

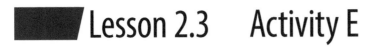 Lesson 2.3   Activity E

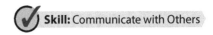 **Skill:** Communicate with Others

Communicating with Your Doctor

Instructions: *Communicating clearly and effectively with your healthcare providers is an important part of receiving healthcare. Read the following scenarios and imagine that you are the patient. Clearly communicate your issue and write questions that will allow you to obtain valuable information for your health issue.*

Scenario 1

Most days, you feel worried from the time you wake up. You tell your guardians this, and they ask what is worrying you. The confusing part is that you are unsure where the worry comes from. You are not stressed about your schoolwork or your job with student government. You are not fighting with any of your friends. You have no reason to be worried, but you cannot shake that feeling.

1. Describe to the doctor how you are feeling.

_____

_____

_____

2. List three or more questions you could ask your doctor to learn more about the issue and lessen the severity.

_____

_____

_____

_____

_____

Scenario 2

You have pimples and whiteheads on your face and chest. You ask your older brother what you can do, and he tells you to start washing your face before going to sleep. You do, and you even go to the store and buy a special face wash, but the pimples do not go away. You feel so self-conscious at school about people looking at you, but you do not know what else you can do.

1. Describe to the doctor how you are feeling.

_____

_____

_____

2. List three or more questions you could ask your doctor to learn more about the issue and lessen the severity.

_____

_____

_____

_____

_____

Name _____ Date _____ Period _____

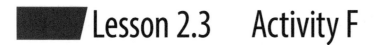 Lesson 2.3   Activity F

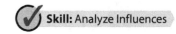

Getting Needed Healthcare

Instructions: *Read the following scenarios and answer the questions about the influences that affect whether each teen accesses needed health services.*

Scenario 1

> Sophia has not been to the doctor's office in years. Luckily, she does not often get sick with more than a simple cold. Her parents told her that if she is not sick, she has no reason to visit the doctor. She thinks her hearing and vision are fine because she has never needed to have them tested. Sophia is not certain about whether she has received all of her vaccinations.

1. What factors influence Sophia's decision to not visit her doctor?

   _____

   _____

2. Should Sophia visit the doctor even if she is not sick? Why or why not?

   _____

   _____

Scenario 2

> Last year, Elijah's doctor diagnosed him with bipolar disorder. His family initially was supportive in getting him the treatment he needed, and he started attending therapy and taking medication. Elijah's dad, however, was recently laid off from his job. Without his dad's company health insurance, Elijah's family cannot afford to continue his treatment.

1. What factors influence Elijah's ability to access health services?

   _____

   _____

2. What can Elijah and his family do to get the services he needs?

   _____

   _____

Scenario 3

> Since Joselyn started swimming for her high school team, she has experienced tendinitis in her shoulder. Initially, Joselyn's coach told her to rest and ice her shoulder. The pain has recently gotten so bad that Joselyn could not compete in her swim meet. Her coach says she needs physical therapy to help her overcome this tendinitis, but the closest clinic is an hour and a half away.

1. What factors influence Joselyn's ability to access health services?

   _____

   _____

2. What can Joselyn and her family do to get the services she needs?

   _____

   _____

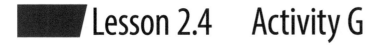 Lesson 2.4   Activity G

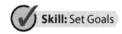

Your Impact on Your Community

Instructions: *Set a SMART goal to improve the community health of your hometown. Answer the following questions to help you achieve your objective.*

1. In what areas would you like to see improvement in your community?

   _____

   _____

   _____

2. Create a central goal to achieve this objective.

   _____

   _____

3. To be sure your goal is SMART, indicate how it meets each of the following.

   A. Specific: _____

   B. Measurable: _____

   C. Achievable: _____

   D. Relevant: _____

   E. Timely: _____

4. List three short-term goals that will help you on your way to achieving your larger goal.

   A. Goal: _____

   _____

   B. Goal: _____

   _____

   C. Goal: _____

   _____

5. Name one obstacle that might stop you from achieving your goal. How can you overcome this obstacle?

   _____

   _____

   _____

   _____

   _____

   _____

   _____

6. Whom can you reach out to for help or support in going after your goal?

   _____

   _____

   _____

Name _____ Date _____ Period _____

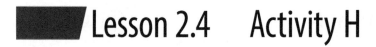 Lesson 2.4 Activity H

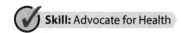

Promoting the Health of Your Community

Instructions: *There are countless opportunities to provide community service through volunteering. Sometimes, it is difficult to know how to start. Answer the following questions to piece together a volunteer opportunity in your community.*

1. List five volunteer opportunities that are available in your local community.

   A. Opportunity: _____

   B. Opportunity: _____

   C. Opportunity: _____

   D. Opportunity: _____

   E. Opportunity: _____

2. Select one opportunity that appeals to you. Which one did you choose and why?

   _____

   _____

   _____

   _____

Instructions: *Find more information about this volunteer opportunity. Use their website if they have one, or contact someone at the organization that provides the community service.*

3. What services does this volunteer opportunity provide?

   _____

   _____

   _____

4. What kind of volunteers is this opportunity looking for? Do you need any qualifications to volunteer with this organization? If yes, list them.

   _____

   _____

   _____

   _____

5. When does this volunteer opportunity take place?

   _____

   _____

6. Where does this volunteer opportunity take place? How would you get there?

   _____

   _____

7. How can you sign up to volunteer?

   _____

   _____

Chapter 2   Activity I

Practice Test

Completion

Instructions: *Write the term that completes the statement in the space provided.*

1. Working with others to make a decision is called _____ decision-making.

_____

2. The ability to locate, interpret, and apply information pertaining to your health is called health _____.

_____

3. A(n) _____ is someone who purchases goods and services.

_____

4. The _____ Service of the United States Department of Health and Human Services provides leadership, funding, and oversight of the healthcare system.

_____

5. A(n) _____ is an area without nearby full-service grocery stores.

_____

True/False

Instructions: *Indicate whether each statement below is true or false.*

6. _____ *True or false?* Failing to achieve a goal you have set does not benefit you.

7. _____ *True or false?* Reliable health information can usually be found on websites with URL stems of .gov, .edu, and .org.

8. _____ *True or false?* The size or popularity of a newspaper or magazine is a good indicator of how much you can trust the information it provides.

9. _____ *True or false?* The healthcare field employs more people than any other type of business in the United States.

10. _____ *True or false?* People living in highly populated areas are exposed to more air and water pollution.

Multiple Choice

Instructions: *Select the letter that corresponds to the correct answer.*

11. _____ Which of the following goals is SMART?
     A. Put away digital devices 30 minutes before bed every night this week.
     B. Get a role in the school musical.
     C. Reduce stress.
     D. Eat more fruits and vegetables and drink more water.

12. _____ Which of the following is true about the theories and health claims resulting from pseudoscience?
     A. They are based on experimentation and observation.
     B. They are peer-reviewed.
     C. They are based on experiment results that cannot be repeated.
     D. They are verified by other scientists.

13. _____ A type of healthcare professional who can deliver health services, but who works under the supervision of primary care physicians, is a(n) _____.
     A. osteopathic doctor
     B. specialist
     C. nurse
     D. physician assistant

14. _____ Which of the following community resources connects people to mental health professionals who can help them seek treatment?

    A. older adult services

    B. community centers

    C. crisis hotlines

    D. All of the above.

Matching

Instructions: *Match each key term to its definition (15–19).*

15. _____ healthcare facilities in which patients reside for the duration of treatment

16. _____ qualities or priorities one considers important

17. _____ healthcare professionals who have additional training in treating certain types of diseases and disorders

18. _____ to take actions that show support

19. _____ area without nearby full-service grocery stores

    A. advocate

    B. food desert

    C. inpatient facilities

    D. specialists

    E. values

Analyzing Data

Instructions: *Read the following data from the US Government Information on Organ Donation and Transplantation. Use the information provided to answer the following questions.*

Another person in the US joins the national organ transplant waiting list every 10 minutes. Each day, about 80 people receive organ transplants.

Organ	Kidney	Liver	Heart	Lung	Other
Percent of total number of people on the waiting list	83.7%	11.6%	3.3%	1.2%	1.5%
Percent of transplants performed	57.9%	22.6%	9.33%	6.9%	3.2%

US Government Information on Organ Donation and Transplantation

Figure 1. US Government Information on Organ Donation and Transplantation

20. There were 36,518 organ transplants performed in 2018. How many heart transplants were performed?

_____

21. At the current rate, how many people will join the organ transplant waiting list each hour? each day? each year?

_____

_____

22. What do you think communities and organizations can do to encourage people to register to become organ donors?

_____

_____

_____

Short Answer

Instructions: *Answer the following questions using what you have learned in this chapter.*

23. Explain the difference between science and pseudoscience.

_____

_____

24. List three questions examined in environmental justice.

_____

_____

_____

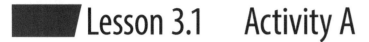

CHAPTER 3 **Interpersonal Skills**

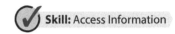

Lesson 3.1   Activity A

Skill: Access Information

Cultural Communication Differences

Instructions: *Using reliable sources, research three cultural communication differences and record your findings. Then, answer the questions below.*

Research Findings

1. List a cultural communication difference: _____

   A. Verbal or nonverbal: _____

   B. Example of a situation in which this might occur: _____

   _____

   C. Provide a source of information: _____

2. List a cultural communication difference: _____

   A. Verbal or nonverbal: _____

   B. Example of a situation in which this might occur: _____

   _____

   C. Provide a source of information: _____

3. List a cultural communication difference: _____

   A. Verbal or nonverbal: _____

   B. Example of a situation in which this might occur: _____

   _____

   C. Provide a source of information: _____

Questions

1. Give an example of how people might be able to overcome cultural communication difference #1.

   _____

   _____

2. Give an example of how people might be able to overcome cultural communication difference #2.

   _____

   _____

3. Give an example of how people might be able to overcome cultural communication difference #3.

   _____

   _____

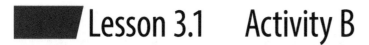 Lesson 3.1   Activity B

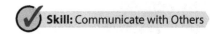 **Skill:** Communicate with Others

Being Assertive in a Relationship

Instructions: *The best communication style for building healthy relationships is assertive communication. Effective assertive communication uses I-statements to express feelings and desires in a respectful manner. Reference the textbook to review the use of I-statements. Respond to the following scenarios in a respectful, assertive way using I-statements.*

1. Your best friend made the show choir and you did not.
   A. What I-statement would you use to respond?

   _____

2. A group of your closest friends goes to the movies and does not invite you.
   A. What I-statement would you use to respond?

   _____

3. Reviewing your grade on your paper, you disagree with your teacher's decision.
   A. What I-statement would you use to respond?

   _____

4. Your dating partner keeps asking if you are ready to have sex.
   A. What I-statement would you use to respond?

   _____

5. Your friend comments "jokes" on your social media post that hurt your feelings.
   A. What I-statement would you use to respond?

   _____

6. After a long and stressful day, your dad asks you to start on your list of chores right away.
   A. What I-statement would you use to respond?

   _____

7. Since you and your best friend started going to different high schools, you feel ignored and lonely.
   A. What I-statement would you use to respond?

   _____

8. You feel like your parents are putting a lot of pressure on you to go to a good college, which creates anxiety.
   A. What I-statement would you use to respond?

   _____

9. The mom of the kids you babysit offers to drive you home. She has been out drinking tonight.
   A. What I-statement would you use to respond?

   _____

Name _____ Date _____ Period _____

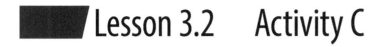 Lesson 3.2   Activity C

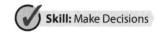

Resolving Conflict

Instructions: *Conflict is a normal part of everyday life, and it is not always bad. Engaging in conflict can have positive outcomes for yourself and your relationships. For each scenario described below, explain how a resolution might be achieved. Use the strategies discussed in the lesson to decide how to resolve the conflict.*

Scenario 1

> Vincent's friend Jamie is having a party on Saturday. Vincent knows, however, that his parents think Jamie is a negative influence and will not let him go. Jamie drinks alcohol and occasionally skips classes at school. When Vincent approaches his parents about attending the party, they tell him that they will not discuss the matter and that they do not want Vincent to interact with Jamie outside of school. Vincent gets angry and goes to his bedroom, slamming the door.

1. What can Vincent and his parents do to resolve this conflict?

_____

_____

_____

_____

_____

_____

_____

_____

_____

Scenario 2

> Mariska and Will have been dating for a year. Mariska is involved in several extracurricular organizations and activities, and she finds it hard to spend quality time with Will as well as her friends with her hectic schedule. One afternoon, Will tells Mariska that he is not happy with the way their relationship has been going. He irritably delivers an ultimatum: "You have to reevaluate your priorities, or I will break up with you."

1. What can Will and Mariska do to resolve this conflict?

_____

_____

_____

_____

_____

_____

_____

_____

_____

Scenario 3

Steve and Jack are in the same trigonometry class. While Jack is doing exceptionally well in trigonometry, Steve has been frustrated attempting to understand the material. Because Steve sits next to Jack in class, he asks Jack to let him copy his answers to the test questions. Jack replies, "Are you serious? I'm not jeopardizing my college scholarship so you can cheat, idiot." Steve angrily tells his friend, "Thanks a lot. I'd help you out if you needed it."

1. What can Steve and Jack do to resolve this conflict?

_____

_____

_____

_____

_____

_____

_____

_____

Scenario 4

Zuri's parents have asked her to babysit her baby sister on Saturday so they can go out for a date night for the first time in months. Zuri explains that the boy she likes at school has finally asked her for a date—on Saturday night. She is concerned that if she cancels the date, she will not be asked out again. "I always get stuck babysitting," Zuri complains.

1. What can Zuri and her parents do to resolve this conflict?

_____

_____

_____

_____

_____

_____

_____

_____

Name _____ Date _____ Period _____

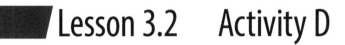 Lesson 3.2   Activity D   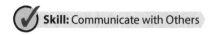 Skill: Communicate with Others

What Would You Do and Say?

Instructions: *Imagine that you are in the following scenarios. Respond to the scenarios by indicating what you would do and say to resolve the conflict respectfully and effectively.*

1. A rumor spread around school that I got alcohol poisoning at a party and almost died. It wasn't true at all, and it hurt that so many people believed it. To make things worse, the person who started the rumor is someone I thought was a friend.

   A. What would you do? _____

   _____

   B. What would you say? _____

   _____

2. I'm tired of my mom always getting into my business. She constantly asks who I'm texting and doesn't let me have any privacy. Yesterday, I asked if I could get a lock for my bedroom door. She said "no" without even hearing me out. I feel very angry.

   A. What would you do? _____

   _____

   B. What would you say? _____

   _____

3. Tyasia is my best friend. Lately, she has been hanging out with a new group of kids at school and seems to ignore me when I am around. I'm really hurt. If this is how she is going to treat me, she can find a new ride to school.

   A. What would you do? _____

   _____

   B. What would you say? _____

   _____

4. Elliott and I have been dating for three months. One day, I saw a flirty text on his phone from another girl. I asked who was texting him, and he said it was just one of his buddies. I am mad.

   A. What would you do? _____

   _____

   B. What would you say? _____

   _____

5. During soccer practice, Jen and I bumped into each other pretty hard. Jen yelled at me, so I yelled back. Jen whispered that she was going to beat me up after practice.

   A. What would you do? _____

   _____

   B. What would you say? _____

   _____

Name _____ Date _____ Period _____

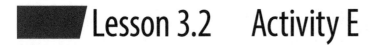

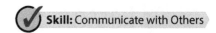

Responding to Conflicts

Instructions: *Your response to conflict can escalate or de-escalate a situation. Often when conflict arises, angry words are spoken. Indicate how you could respond to each statement in a respectful and assertive way that de-escalates the situation and begins the conversation to resolve the conflict.*

1. A teammate says to you after practice, "You need to stop cheating, or I'll tell Coach."

   A. How would you respond?

   _____

   _____

   _____

2. A friend tells you, "You haven't texted me back in days! If you don't want to be friends anymore, just tell me."

   A. How would you respond?

   _____

   _____

   _____

3. A classmate corners you by your locker and accuses, "I heard you've been talking about me."

   A. How would you respond?

   _____

   _____

   _____

4. Your friend's parents had an emergency pop up, so you drive your friend home for them. You get home past curfew and your guardian tells you that you are grounded.

   A. How would you respond?

   _____

   _____

   _____

5. Think of a recent conflict you had with a person that escalated into anger. Describe the situation. What did you say or could have said to de-escalate the intensity of the conflict?

   _____

   _____

   _____

   _____

   _____

   _____

   _____

   _____

   _____

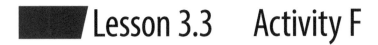 **Lesson 3.3   Activity F**

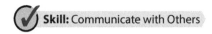 **Skill:** Communicate with Others

Positive and Negative Peer Pressure

Instructions: *Read the following scenarios to determine if the peer pressure being demonstrated is positive or negative. Then, decide how to respond based on the strategies discussed in the textbook.*

1. A teammate encourages you to put your phone away and go to sleep the night before a game.
   A. Is this peer pressure positive or negative?

   _____

   B. How would you respond?

   _____

   _____

   _____

   _____

2. A dating partner begs you to send a nude photo of yourself.
   A. Is this peer pressure positive or negative?

   _____

   B. How would you respond?

   _____

   _____

   _____

   _____

3. A friend tries to convince you to sneak out of your house to hang out late at night.
   A. Is this peer pressure positive or negative?

   _____

   B. How would you respond?

   _____

   _____

   _____

   _____

4. After teasing someone else for not drinking, a friend turns to you to offer you alcohol.
   A. Is this peer pressure positive or negative?

   _____

   B. How would you respond?

   _____

   _____

   _____

   _____

5. Your best friend tries to persuade you to resolve a conflict with your parents.

   A. Is this peer pressure positive or negative?

   _____

   B. How would you respond?

   _____

   _____

   _____

   _____

6. Your sister asked you to lie to your parents about where she was yesterday.

   A. Is this peer pressure positive or negative?

   _____

   B. How would you respond?

   _____

   _____

   _____

   _____

7. After you say no several times, a classmate continues to ask for your homework to copy.

   A. Is this peer pressure positive or negative?

   _____

   B. How would you respond?

   _____

   _____

   _____

   _____

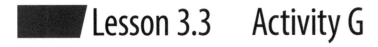 Lesson 3.3   Activity G

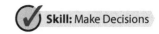 **Skill:** Make Decisions

Resisting Pressure

Instructions: *As a teen, you may feel pressured to join others in risky behaviors. Read the following scenarios and help the teens resist negative pressure and make a good decision by identifying the decision, exploring the alternatives, and selecting the best option by weighing the pros and cons of each one.*

Scenario 1

> Sarah has had a crush on Jordon for months. Recently, he seems to be showing interest in return. Jordon offers to have his friend drive Sarah home with them so she does not have to ride the bus. When Jordon's friend pulls into the parking lot, there are already five of their classmates piled in to the four available passengers' seats. No one is wearing seat belts. Nervous, Sarah jokes that there is not enough space for her. Jordon teases her by saying, "Oh come on, it's only a few miles to your house. Plus, carpooling is good for the environment. Sit on my lap!" Sarah has already missed the bus, and she does not want to disappoint Jordon.

1. What is Sarah's issue or problem? Please describe.

   _____

   _____

   _____

2. List two of Sarah's choices in this situation. What are the pros and cons of each choice?

   A. Choice 1: _____

   _____

   Pros: _____

   _____

   Cons: _____

   _____

   B. Choice 2: _____

   _____

   Pros: _____

   _____

   Cons: _____

   _____

3. Based on the pros and cons, which decision should Sarah make? Defend your decision.

   _____

   _____

   _____

   _____

   _____

   _____

Scenario 2

Peter and a group of friends are hanging out at the mall on Saturday afternoon. Peter likes a shirt he sees in a store, but cannot afford it. Peter's friends dare him to steal it. He just recently started spending time with this group of friends, and Peter wants to impress them so they will let him keep hanging out with them. Peter stole a candy bar once before and got away with it. Tucking the shirt into his pocket, Peter hesitates.

1. What is Peter's issue or problem? Please describe.

   _____

   _____

   _____

2. List two of Peter's choices in this situation. What are the pros and cons of each choice?

   A. Choice 1: _____

      _____

      Pros: _____

      _____

      Cons: _____

      _____

   B. Choice 2: _____

      _____

      Pros: _____

      _____

      Cons: _____

      _____

3. Based on the pros and cons, which decision should Peter make? Defend your decision.

   _____

   _____

   _____

   _____

   _____

   _____

   _____

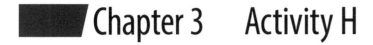 Chapter 3   Activity H

Practice Test

Completion

Instructions: *Write the term that completes the statement in the space provided.*

1. Eye contact is a form of _____ communication.

    _____

2. _____ communication hides or does not clearly state a person's needs, wants, and feelings.

    _____

3. When people _____, they work together to think and talk through a solution to a conflict.

    _____

4. Serious or difficult conflicts can benefit from a neutral _____ to help the conflicting parties reach an agreement.

    _____

5. Outside actions, words, and rewards that influence your behavior are called _____ pressure.

    _____

True/False

Instructions: *Indicate whether each statement below is true or false.*

6. _____ *True or false?* Effective communication requires active listening skills.

7. _____ *True or false?* Trying to resolve a conflict will destroy a relationship or make the conflict worse.

8. _____ *True or false?* Peer pressure can be both positive and negative.

Multiple Choice

Instructions: *Select the letter that corresponds to the correct answer.*

9. _____ Which of the following examples is a form of verbal communication?
    A. facial expressions   C. volume of voice
    B. social media posts   D. B and C.

10. _____ One way to clearly express your needs and preferences is by _____.
    A. dropping subtle hints
    B. assuming others know how you feel
    C. agreeing with something to avoid conflict
    D. showing respect and seeking clarity

11. _____ When mediators act as neutral third parties, they _____.
    A. ensure one person is heard primarily
    B. make the people involved work to find their own solutions
    C. clarify communication
    D. All of the above.

12. _____ Which of the following is a type of indirect peer pressure?
    A. thinking about what will make you seem cool
    B. people minimizing the risks
    C. people teasing you
    D. people making you doubt yourself

Matching

Instructions: *Match each key term to its definition (13–16).*

13. _____ disagreement or argument that occurs due to differing priorities, values, goals, or needs

14. _____ failure in communication that can lead to conflict

15. _____ constructive response to a message

16. _____ motivation to do an activity or take on certain qualities

A. conflict
B. feedback
C. misunderstanding
D. pressure

Analyzing Data

Instructions: *Read the data below from the PEW Research Center on teen conflict. Use the information provided to answer the following questions.*

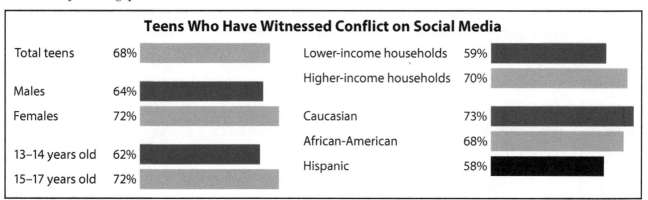

Figure 1. Percentage of teens who have witnessed conflict on social media

17. If 5,000 teens took this survey, how many witnessed conflict on social media? How many did not?

_____

18. What percent more of older teens (15 to 17 years old) witness conflict than younger teens (13 to 14 years old)?

_____

Short Answer

Instructions: *Answer the following questions using what you have learned in this chapter.*

19. List three nonverbal elements that can help reduce misunderstandings in online communication.

_____

_____

_____

_____

_____

20. How can building healthy, respectful relationships help you handle peer pressure?

_____

_____

_____

_____

CHAPTER 4

Promoting Mental and Emotional Health

Lesson 4.1   Activity A

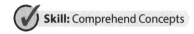

Maslow's Hierarchy of Needs

Instructions: *Fill in the following activity with what you learned about Maslow's hierarchy of human needs in Lesson 4.1. Then respond to the scenario that follows.*

1. Physical Needs

    A. Definition in your own words: _____

    B. Example of a person at this level: _____

2. Security

    A. Definition in your own words: _____

    B. Example of a person at this level: _____

3. Love and Acceptance

    A. Definition in your own words: _____

    B. Example of a person at this level: _____

4. Esteem

    A. Definition in your own words: _____

    B. Example of a person at this level: _____

5. Self-Actualization

    A. Definition in your own words: _____

    B. Example of a person at this level: _____

Scenarios

Instructions: *Read the following scenarios and determine what level of human needs each person or group of people is striving toward.*

1. A teen is bullied at school.

    A. Determine level in Maslow's Hierarchy: _____

2. A teen feels like her family and friends do not truly care about her.

    A. Determine level in Maslow's Hierarchy: _____

3. A teen lives in a neighborhood plagued by violent crime.

    A. Determine level in Maslow's Hierarchy: _____

4. A teen is deciphering what he wants to do after college by considering what makes him passionate.

    A. Determine level in Maslow's Hierarchy: _____

5. A teen who worked hard and got straight As throughout high school hopes to become valedictorian.

    A. Determine level in Maslow's Hierarchy: _____

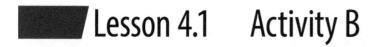 Lesson 4.1   Activity B

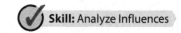   **Skill:** Analyze Influences

Cognitive Distortions

Instructions: *Match each scenario below with the cognitive distortion influencing each person's mental health.*

Scenarios

1. _____ Kim is a straight-A student, but when she gets a bad grade on one exam, she is convinced she will not be able to get into college.

2. _____ Bobby does not often take time to relax. One week, he decides to allow himself a lazy weekend and spends the two days watching television. On Sunday evening, Bobby feels worried that he will always be this lazy.

3. _____ Franco is an average student, but he often thinks about himself in extremes. If he does well on a test, he thinks, "I'm perfect!" If he does badly on a test, however, he thinks he is a failure.

4. _____ Keiko's boyfriend, Mark, is not as neat as she is and does not care about grades as much as she does. She knows this when she begins dating him and intends to make him change.

5. _____ Stephanie is a naturally shy person. When she meets new people, she does not speak with them right away. This often leads people to think that she is stuck-up or does not like them.

6. _____ When Andrew argues with people, he has one goal in mind: winning. Instead of listening to what the other person has to say, he concentrates on what his next response will be.

7. _____ Mallory gets a bad grade on her English paper. Although she spent most of the week watching TV and working on other assignments, Mallory blames the teacher for her bad grade. "She didn't give us enough time," Mallory says.

Cognitive Distortions

A. black-and-white thinking

B. jumping to conclusions

C. catastrophizing

D. control fallacies

E. emotional reasoning

F. fallacy of change

G. always being right

Questions

1. How can cognitive distortions be self-defeating for a person's mental and emotional health?

_____

_____

_____

_____

_____

_____

2. What might you do to challenge these cognitive distortions?

_____

_____

_____

_____

_____

_____

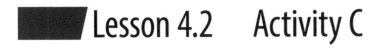 ## Lesson 4.2   Activity C

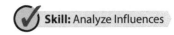

Gender Stereotypes

Instructions: *With a partner, list character traits that are stereotypically associated with each gender within US society. Then, answer the following questions about gender stereotypes.*

1. List masculine traits.

_____

_____

_____

_____

2. List feminine traits.

_____

_____

_____

_____

3. What factors do you think affect the traits a society associates with a gender?

_____

_____

_____

_____

4. People typically have some traits that are societally perceived as masculine and feminine. List at least three masculine characteristics and three feminine characteristics you would associate with yourself.

_____

_____

_____

5. What impact do you think gender stereotypes have on people's concept of their own identity? Explain.

_____

_____

_____

_____

6. Gender stereotypes can negatively influence people's mental and emotional health in many ways. Explain this impact in the following areas.

   A. Internal pressure: _____

   _____

   _____

   B. Social situations: _____

   _____

C. Expectations of gender: _____

_____

_____

D. Success and achievement: _____

_____

_____

E. Interpersonal relationships: _____

_____

_____

F. Conflict and violence: _____

_____

_____

7. What can people do to combat the effects of gender stereotypes? Brainstorm with a group about strategies that individuals, schools, and other organizations can do to help.

_____

_____

_____

_____

_____

_____

_____

_____

_____

_____

_____

_____

_____

_____

_____

_____

_____

_____

_____

_____

_____

_____

_____

Name _____ Date _____ Period _____

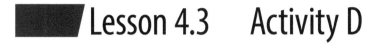
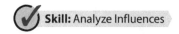 **Skill:** Analyze Influences

Self-Esteem

Instructions: *Read the following stories about Marlen and Lily to learn more about the factors that influence self-esteem and the impact of self-esteem on daily living. Then, answer the questions.*

Marlen's Story

Growing up, Marlen would spent a lot of time at her grandparents' house with her siblings and cousins. She knows from her friends at school that not all siblings get along well, but Marlen has always felt loved and supported by her family. Marlen does not feel any pressure to be perfect or hide mistakes, because her parents taught her that these things make her unique and will help her grow. Marlen wants to prioritize her friendships and schoolwork, so it does not bother her that she has not dated yet. She may not be the fastest swimmer on her team, but she feels proud about how much she has improved personally over the years. Today, Marlen feels good about who she is.

Lily's Story

Lily was bullied throughout grade school. Her classmates mocked her at school, and they never invited her to their birthday parties. Lily's parents just told her to be more friendly and open. When she entered high school, Lily fell in with some older classmates. They often pressure her to do things she is not comfortable with, like vaping or dating an older boy, Jake. She goes along with it because she fears they will stop liking her otherwise. Lily does not believe anyone else at school would like her, so she remains friends with them. She even continues to date Jake, who has recently been disrespectful toward her and pressures her about becoming more intimate.

Questions

1. What factors helped Marlen develop healthy self-esteem? What factors have negatively impacted Lily's self-esteem?

   _____

   _____

   _____

   _____

2. How has Marlen's healthy self-esteem impacted her daily life? How has Lily's low self-esteem impacted her daily life?

   _____

   _____

   _____

   _____

3. What advice would you give to Lily to help her develop healthy self-esteem?

   _____

   _____

   _____

   _____

   _____

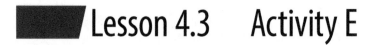 Lesson 4.3   Activity E

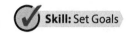 **Skill:** Set Goals

Building Your Self-Esteem

Instructions: *No matter your level of self-esteem, everyone can always take steps to feel more confident about themselves. Answer the following questions and write a SMART goal to improve your self-esteem.*

1. Assess your current level of self-esteem. Do you feel confident in yourself? What areas of your self-esteem can you improve?

   _____

   _____

   _____

   _____

2. How do you want to go about improving your self-esteem? Use at least two different strategies.

   _____

   _____

   _____

   _____

3. How can you track your progress?

   _____

   _____

4. What obstacles might get in your way of achieving this goal? Explain how you can overcome these obstacles.

   _____

   _____

   _____

   _____

   _____

   _____

   _____

   _____

   _____

5. How can you stay on track? How can you stay accountable for your own actions?

   _____

   _____

   _____

   _____

6. Write your SMART goal.

   _____

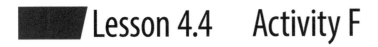 Lesson 4.4   Activity F

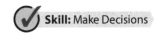 **Skill:** Make Decisions

Emotional Intelligence

Instructions: *Emotional intelligence is a person's skill at perceiving, understanding, and managing emotions and feelings. Rewrite each scenario into a version that depicts each participant making a healthy decision using emotional intelligence.*

Scenario 1

> Since Reagan began dating Hunter, he rarely spends time with his friend Sasha. They used to eat lunch together in the high school cafeteria; now, Reagan usually leaves school to go out for lunch with Hunter. What's more, Reagan rarely replies to her texts. One afternoon, Sasha confronts Reagan after gym class. "What is up with you and Hunter?" she snaps. "Am I not good enough to hang out with you anymore?"

1. Rewrite the scenario showing emotional intelligence.

_____

_____

_____

_____

_____

_____

_____

_____

_____

_____

Scenario 2

> Stephen often does imitations of teachers and classmates, which his friends think are hilarious and spot-on. One morning before class, Stephen is imitating his classmate Jon. When Jon enters the classroom, he notices the students crowded around Stephen. Jon realizes what is happening as one of the other students quickly motions to Stephen to stop. Stephen turns to see Jon walking in and dismissively says, "Hey, I was only joking." Jon, sulking, ignores him.

1. Rewrite the scenario showing emotional intelligence.

_____

_____

_____

_____

_____

_____

_____

_____

_____

Scenario 3

Aisha, a new student at Kennedy High School, has begun to date Alec. Aisha is unaware that Alec recently broke up with Rhiannon, his girlfriend of more than a year. One afternoon during lunch, Rhiannon approaches Aisha and tells her that Alec is bad news and he eventually will "dump" Aisha. Aisha tells Rhiannon to mind her own business. Later, Aisha learns that Rhiannon is still hurt and angry because she felt Alec abruptly broke up with her.

1. Rewrite the scenario showing emotional intelligence.

_____

_____

_____

_____

_____

_____

_____

_____

_____

Scenario 4

Dante and Brody are high school seniors competing for an internship at a prestigious law firm. Dante has worked hard, earning mostly As on top of caring for his younger sister with Down syndrome. Brody has maintained a B-minus average and has a reputation for being the class clown. Shortly after their interviews, Dante is astonished to learn that Brody was selected for the internship. Dante remarks to Brody that "apparently, slackers are 'in' this year."

1. Rewrite the scenario showing emotional intelligence.

_____

_____

_____

_____

_____

_____

_____

_____

_____

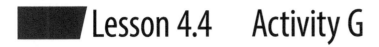 # Lesson 4.4   Activity G

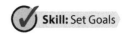

What Is Your EI?

Instructions: *For this activity, assess your emotional intelligence and set a goal toward improving it in the future.*

1. Identify the strengths and weaknesses of your emotional intelligence.

A. Strengths: _____

_____

_____

_____

_____

_____

B. Weaknesses: _____

_____

_____

_____

_____

_____

2. How can improving your emotional intelligence affect your mental and emotional, social, and physical health? Explain.

_____

_____

_____

_____

_____

_____

_____

_____

_____

_____

_____

_____

_____

_____

_____

_____

_____

_____

_____

3. Set goals for improving your emotional intelligence.

   A. Write your overarching SMART goal.

   _____

   _____

   _____

   _____

   _____

   _____

   B. Write smaller goals to break down your SMART goal.

   Goal: _____

   _____

   _____

   _____

   _____

   _____

   Goal: _____

   _____

   _____

   _____

   _____

   _____

   Goal: _____

   _____

   _____

   _____

   _____

   _____

Name _____ Date _____ Period _____

Chapter 4   Activity H

Practice Test

Completion

Instructions: *Write the term that completes the statement in the space provided.*

1. A person with a genetic _____ has an increased risk of developing a health condition due to inherited genes.

   _____

2. The fundamental beliefs and ideals people hold that guide their behaviors and choices are core _____.

   _____

3. Gender _____ are culturally defined assumptions about what it means to be male or female.

   _____

4. Holding yourself to impossibly high standards, called _____, is harmful to self-esteem.

   _____

5. The ability to control one's emotions and impulses and to act with careful deliberation and integrity is called _____.

   _____

True/False

Instructions: *Indicate whether each statement below is true or false.*

6. _____ *True or false?* Mental and emotional health are *not* exclusively positive or negative, but exist on a continuum.

7. _____ *True or false?* Social identity is one's connection to different cultural or ethnic groups.

8. _____ *True or false?* According to Erikson, developing a sense of personal identity is the primary task of adolescence.

9. _____ *True or false?* Self-esteem is your mental picture of yourself, including your appearance, skills and abilities, and weaknesses.

10. _____ *True or false?* People with high emotional intelligence are skilled at understanding the emotions of others.

Multiple Choice

Instructions: *Select the letter that corresponds to the correct answer.*

11. _____ A mental _____ is when feelings that decrease mental health temporarily impair a person's ability to cope with daily life.
    A. health condition
    B. distress
    C. illness
    D. disorder

12. _____ Which of the following is the combination of thoughts, feelings, and behaviors that make you unique?
    A. core value
    B. social identity
    C. personality
    D. ethnicity

13. _____ Which of the following is a characteristic of people with healthy self-esteem?
    A. attempt new activities and embrace challenges
    B. make decisions to avoid rejection
    C. are sensitive to criticism
    D. view negative events as failures

14. _____ Which defense mechanism means explaining or making excuses for your bad behavior?
    A. intellectualization
    B. reaction formation
    C. rationalization
    D. displacement

Matching

Instructions: *Match each key term to its definition (15–21).*

15. _____ characteristics and qualities that distinguish who a person is

16. _____ mental picture of one's abilities, appearance, and personality based on experiences and interactions with others

17. _____ skill in perceiving, understanding, and managing emotions and feelings

18. _____ confidence in one's own worth and abilities

19. _____ feeling of reaching one's full potential through creativity, independence, spontaneity, and a grasp of the real world

20. _____ one's connection to a particular social group that shares similar cultural or national ties

21. _____ preconceived ideas, roles, and characteristics people associate with a certain gender

A. emotional intelligence
B. ethnicity
C. gender stereotypes
D. identity
E. self-actualization
F. self-esteem
G. self-image

Analyzing Data

Instructions: *The following chart presents the percentage of the US population who have completed four years of college or more between 1978 and 2018. Use the information provided to answer the following questions.*

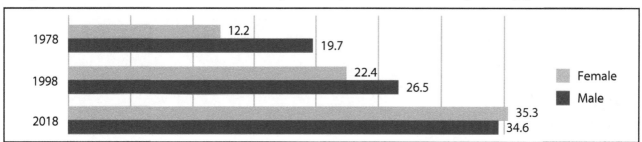

US Census Bureau

Figure 1. Percentage of the US population who have completed four years of college or more

22. What is the difference in the percent of females who completed four years of college or more in 1978 and 2018? in the percent of males?

_____

23. What factors do you think have impacted these increases to college attendance? What role do you think shifts in gender stereotypes has played?

_____

_____

_____

Short Answer

Instructions: *Answer the following questions using what you have learned in this chapter.*

24. What are some common traits of people with positive mental and emotional health?

_____

_____

25. Explain how social media can be either a protective factor or a risk factor for mental and emotional health.

_____

_____

_____

CHAPTER 5   Shifting to Positive Thinking

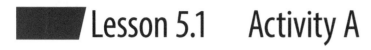 Lesson 5.1   Activity A   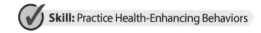 **Skill:** Practice Health-Enhancing Behaviors

Give a Little, Get a Lot

Instructions: *Giving to other people increases happiness, improves health, and may extend lives. This can include big donations and volunteer operations or simple, free acts of kindness. For one week, make it your mission to give something to another person every day. Create a table like the one below to keep track, and answer the questions that follow.*

Day of the Week	Form of Giving	Recipient(s)	Time Required	Money Required
Sunday	Listening to my friends	Best friend	One hour	None

Figure 1. Giving table

1. Was it difficult to come up with ideas for how to give to others? Explain.

   _____

   _____

   _____

   _____

   _____

   _____

2. What was your favorite action from this week? How did it make you feel to do this for another person?

   _____

   _____

   _____

   _____

   _____

   _____

3. Which of these actions would you be happy to do again? Explain.

   _____

   _____

   _____

   _____

   _____

   _____

Name _____ Date _____ Period _____

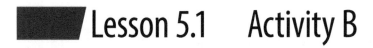 Lesson 5.1   Activity B

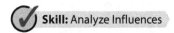

Influencing Happiness

Instructions: *Read the following scenarios and answer the questions about the influences that affect a teen's happiness.*

Scenario 1

Juanita has many friends from childhood, but she is still a little nervous about making new friends in high school. Her dad and brother are both shy, introverted people who do not socialize very often. When Juanita asked her mom about it, she said, "Well, I had a friend who betrayed me in high school so it's not even worth the effort."

1. What factor primarily influences Juanita's happiness in this scenario? Explain.

_____

_____

2. Does this factor mean Juanita cannot change her level of happiness? Why or why not?

_____

_____

Scenario 2

Henry feels like he is living his life for other people. His parents expect him to become the first person in his family to go to college, and he wants to make them happy. So he works hard at school, and even joins the Latin club as an extracurricular activity. Henry gets upset when he fails something because he feels like he is letting his parents down. Henry sees kids in his class who are passionate about their activities or the colleges they apply to, and Henry does not feel excited about it. He feels a bit like he is just going through the motions.

1. What factor primarily influences Henry's happiness in this scenario? Explain.

_____

_____

2. What can Henry do to increase his happiness?

_____

Scenario 3

Charlotte loves her parents, but she never really sees them. As a lawyer and a nurse, her parents regularly work long hours. As soon as she was old enough, Charlotte's parents allowed her to take care of herself before and after school. Charlotte does not have many friends at school. She never knows what to say in social situations, so she remains quiet. She feels like no one really knows her, and she is never sure who to turn to for help when she has an issue.

1. What factor primarily influences Charlotte's happiness in this scenario?

_____

_____

2. How can this factor affect Charlotte's physical health?

_____

_____

Name _____ Date _____ Period _____

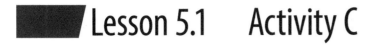 Lesson 5.1   Activity C

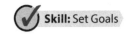

Adopting Healthy Behaviors

Instructions: *Setting and working toward goals can help increase your sense of happiness. The same is true of engaging in simple, healthy behaviors like getting enough sleep, being physically active, spending time in nature, or eating nutritious foods. Answer the following questions to set a SMART goal to increase happiness.*

1. In small groups, brainstorm simple, healthy behaviors that increase happiness.

_____

_____

_____

_____

_____

_____

_____

2. Create a central goal to implement one of these ideas to improve happiness.

_____

_____

3. To be sure your goal is SMART, indicate how it meets each of the following.

    A. Specific: _____

    B. Measurable: _____

    C. Achievable: _____

    D. Relevant: _____

    E. Timely: _____

4. List three short-term goals that will help you achieve your central goal.

    A. Goal: _____

    _____

    B. Goal: _____

    _____

    C. Goal: _____

    _____

5. How will you keep yourself accountable for achieving this goal?

_____

_____

_____

6. Whom can you reach out to for help or support in going after your goal?

_____

_____

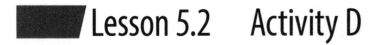 Lesson 5.2   Activity D

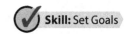

Improving Your Mind-Set

Instructions: *You learned many strategies for pursuing a positive mind-set in Lesson 5.2. Answer the following questions to set a SMART goal to improve or maintain your positive mind-set.*

1. Assess your current general mind-set. What do you do well? What could you do better?

   _____

   _____

2. Identify a basic goal for maintaining or improving your positive mind-set.

   _____

3. State what you would like to achieve. Be **specific**.

   _____

4. How will you measure whether or not you have **achieved** this goal?

   _____

5. Set short-term goals to help make your large goal more **achievable**.

   _____

   _____

   _____

6. How is this goal **relevant** to your current identity and values?

   _____

   _____

7. Set a reasonable **time line** for completing your goal. Set dates for your short-term goals as well as your larger goal.

   _____

   _____

8. How will you act on this goal? Whom will you ask for support?

   _____

   _____

9. How will you monitor your progress?

   _____

10. What obstacles might keep you from reaching your goal? How can you overcome these obstacles?

    _____

    _____

11. Summarize the information from these questions as your comprehensive SMART goal.

    _____

    _____

    _____

    _____

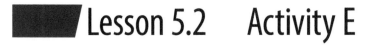 Lesson 5.2   Activity E

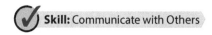 **Skill:** Communicate with Others

Making Better Self-Talk

Instructions: *Read the following examples of negative self-talk which can undermine confidence and motivation. Rewrite each example with a statement of positive self-talk. This statement should be encouraging and supportive. Practice saying these positive statements aloud to yourself or with a partner.*

1. Statement of negative self-talk: Why bother studying for this test? I'm terrible at history, and I know I'm going to fail.

   A. Statement of positive self-talk: _____

   _____

2. Statement of negative self-talk: I'm short and slow. I'll never make the volleyball team, no matter how hard I try.

   A. Statement of positive self-talk: _____

   _____

3. Statement of negative self-talk: I hate the way I look in pictures. I wish I looked like my friends do on social media.

   A. Statement of positive self-talk: _____

   _____

4. Statement of negative self-talk: I'm so upset about losing the championship game and I'll never feel better.

   A. Statement of positive self-talk: _____

   _____

5. Statement of negative self-talk: I can't speak to new people without embarrassing myself. Who would want to date me?

   A. Statement of positive self-talk: _____

   _____

6. Statement of negative self-talk: My friends passed their driver's tests on the first try, but I've failed it twice. I'm so stupid.

   A. Statement of positive self-talk: _____

   _____

7. Statement of negative self-talk: I'm so awkward and weird and nobody likes me. What's wrong with me?

   A. Statement of positive self-talk: _____

   _____

8. Statement of negative self-talk: I always do terribly on tests, so I'm going to tank the ACT for sure.

   A. Statement of positive self-talk: _____

   _____

9. Statement of negative self-talk: My friends all hate me; that's why they aren't texting me back.

   A. Statement of positive self-talk: _____

   _____

Name _____ Date _____ Period _____

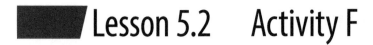 Lesson 5.2   Activity F   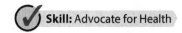 **Skill:** Advocate for Health

Advocating for Respect

Instructions: *Part of adopting a positive mind-set is having respect for other people who may have different backgrounds, experiences, and perspectives from you. Promote respect for diversity in your community by speaking to a specific target audience. To help you organize your message, answer the following questions.*

1. Select a target audience (a specific part of your community).

   _____

2. Why is respecting diversity important? What benefits does it have for people in your community?

   _____

   _____

   _____

   _____

3. Assess your target audience's current practices in regards to respecting diversity. What does your audience do well? What can it do better?

   _____

   _____

   _____

   _____

   _____

   _____

4. What strategies can your audience implement to respect other people better? List at least three.

   _____

   _____

   _____

   _____

   _____

   _____

   _____

5. What can your audience do to encourage others to respect diversity too?

   _____

   _____

   _____

   _____

   _____

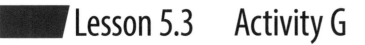 # Lesson 5.3   Activity G

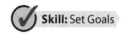

Set a Goal toward Empathy

Instructions: *Read the following scenarios and write a long-term SMART goal that can help each person build empathy. Then, write two short-term goals that will help break up this long-term goal into more manageable pieces.*

Scenario 1

Rashaud's friend comes to him about a fight she is having with her foster mom. While she explains, Rashaud jumps in to say, "Moms are the worst, aren't they?" He goes on to tell a story about a conflict he had with his mom the month before. Rashaud's friend patiently waits for him to finish his story and then says, "I can see how that would be frustrating." She does not ask Rashaud what she should do with her foster mom. She really just wanted to vent to someone who cares. Rashaud, however, explains that he knows how she can fix this issue.

1. Long-term goal: _____

2. Short-term goals: _____

_____

_____

_____

Scenario 2

Camila is considering quitting the US Politics Club at school. She gets so frustrated at each meeting hearing values so contrary to hers. She wonders how anyone can have those opinions when her perspective is clearly more logical. The faculty moderator for the club starts each meeting by reminding everyone to keep an open mind and not judge any stances, but Camila thinks some opinions are just wrong. She does not understand where other people's perspectives come from sometimes.

1. Long-term goal: _____

2. Short-term goals: _____

_____

_____

_____

Scenario 3

Jimmy's dating partner gets angry with him sometimes because he does not seem to listen, but Jimmy thinks he is just a good multitasker. His partner suggests an activity for their next date night while Jimmy checks the notifications on his phone. He sees that he got a new message from his teammate asking about game times and he shoots back a response. When he looks back up, Jimmy's partner asks him, "Did you hear anything I just said?"

1. Long-term goal: _____

2. Short-term goals: _____

_____

_____

_____

Name _____ Date _____ Period _____

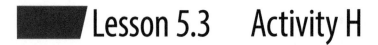 Lesson 5.3   Activity H

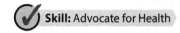 **Skill:** Advocate for Health

Helping Others Build Resilience

Instructions: *Answer the following questions and create an advocacy campaign that teaches peers at your school about building resilience.*

1. What is resilience to you?

_____

_____

2. Do some people naturally have more resilience than others? Can people build resilience? Explain.

_____

_____

_____

3. What are the benefits of having resilience throughout life?

_____

_____

_____

_____

_____

4. With a partner, brainstorm some strategies for building resilience. Use the strategies from Lesson 5.3 for help.

_____

_____

_____

_____

_____

_____

_____

_____

_____

_____

5. What do you think is the best way to get this information across to other students at your school? Select one medium and explain your choice.

_____

_____

_____

_____

_____

Instructions: *Implement this campaign in the medium of your choice.*

Name _____ Date _____ Period _____

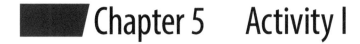 **Chapter 5   Activity I**

Practice Test

Completion

Instructions: *Write the term that completes the statement in the space provided.*

1. The belief that a person's most basic abilities and feelings are permanent is called a(n) _____ mind-set.

   _____

2. A state of _____ is a state of concentrated, judgment-free awareness of what is happening in the present moment.

   _____

3. Showing appreciation for what you have, or _____, can help give people a more positive mind-set.

   _____

4. The ability to experience the emotions another person is feeling is _____ empathy.

   _____

5. _____ can help people adapt well even when facing difficult circumstances.

   _____

True/False

Instructions: *Indicate whether each statement below is true or false.*

6. _____ *True or false?* The biggest predictor of life satisfaction is the quality of a person's relationships.

7. _____ *True or false?* Even optimistic people view situations negatively when faced with challenges.

8. _____ *True or false?* You can only directly control situations and events within your Field of Influence.

9. _____ *True or false?* People with resilience see moments of change as opportunities for growth and new experiences.

Multiple Choice

Instructions: *Write the letter that corresponds to the correct answer in the blank space.*

10. _____ Which of the following is a character trait influenced by genes?
    A. optimism   C. resilience
    B. outgoingness   D. All of the above

11. _____ Which of the following situations is within a person's Field of Control?
    A. getting enough sleep   C. what other people think or say
    B. making a new friend   D. past mistakes

12. _____ People with empathy _____.
    A. rush to find solutions to challenges
    B. ask questions to clarify others' feelings
    C. judge or blame people for challenges
    D. None of the above.

Matching

Instructions: *Match each key term to its definition (13–18).*

13. _____ ability to understand and share the feelings of another person

14. _____ act of thinking deeply or obsessively about negative feelings or situations

15. _____ way of thinking or feeling about a situation

16. _____ person's thought pattern, attitude, and mood

17. _____ ability to recover from traumatic and stressful events

18. _____ stable and generalized intention to accomplish something that is both meaningful to the self and consequential for the world beyond the self

A. empathy
B. mind-set
C. outlook
D. purpose
E. resilience
F. rumination

Analyzing Data

Instructions: *The following chart shows information from the 2019 World Happiness Report. Use the information provided to answer the following questions.*

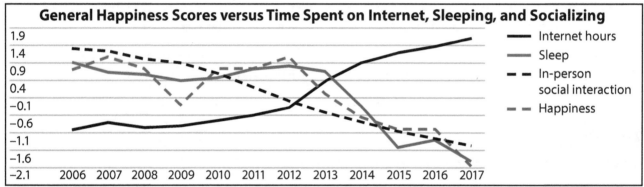

Figure 2. General happiness scores in relation to time spent on the Internet, sleeping, and socializing

19. What has been the general trend of happiness over the last five years?

_____

20. What has been the trend for in-person social interactions? What impact do you think this has had on overall happiness?

_____

_____

21. What can people do to increase their happiness rates?

_____

_____

Short Answer

Instructions: *Answer the following questions using what you have learned in this chapter.*

22. What impact can self-respect have on a person's mind-set?

_____

_____

23. Compare and contrast cognitive empathy and emotional empathy.

_____

_____

Managing the Stress in Your Life

Lesson 6.1   Activity A

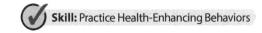 **Skill:** Practice Health-Enhancing Behaviors

Acute Versus Chronic Stress

Instructions: *For this activity, review the stressors below and categorize the stressors as acute or chronic. Then, add five stressors you have experienced in your own life. Identify whether these stressors are acute or chronic.*

1. Your family is moving to a new state next week.

   A. Is this stressor acute or chronic? _____

2. Your teacher gives you only four days to complete an important project.

   A. Is this stressor acute or chronic? _____

3. At 10:00 p.m. the night before your biology final, you don't feel prepared.

   A. Is this stressor acute or chronic? _____

4. Your mother announces that she is pregnant.

   A. Is this stressor acute or chronic? _____

5. You realize your sister took your favorite jeans.

   A. Is this stressor acute or chronic? _____

6. Your best friend tagged an embarrassing picture of you online.

   A. Is this stressor acute or chronic? _____

7. Your parents announce they are getting a divorce.

   A. Is this stressor acute or chronic? _____

8. You text the group chat something you meant to send to only one friend.

   A. Is this stressor acute or chronic? _____

9. You are waiting in the lobby before your first job interview.

   A. Is this stressor acute or chronic? _____

10. Your grandmother is diagnosed with breast cancer.

    A. Is this stressor acute or chronic? _____

11. Enter your own stressor: _____

    _____

    A. Is this stressor acute or chronic? _____

12. Enter your own stressor: _____

    _____

    A. Is this stressor acute or chronic? _____

13. Enter your own stressor: _____

_____

    A. Is this stressor acute or chronic?_____

14. Enter your own stressor: _____

_____

    A. Is this stressor acute or chronic?_____

15. Enter your own stressor: _____

_____

    A. Is this stressor acute or chronic?_____

16. Choose one stressor and explain how you would reduce or manage your stress in this situation.

_____

_____

_____

_____

_____

_____

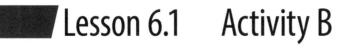 Lesson 6.1   Activity B

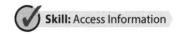

Most Stressful Cities in the US

Instructions: *Several studies have explored the idea that some US cities are more stressful than others. Find one of these studies online and choose four cities that are considered to be the most stressful. Then, identify the stressors that residents of each city face. Finally, identify stressors in your own hometown and describe how your hometown compares to the cities on this list.*

1. Title of study:_____

2. Web source: _____

City Stressors

1. Enter city name: _____

   A. Stress ranking: _____

   B. List the stressors: _____

   _____

   _____

   _____

2. Enter city name: _____

   A. Stress ranking: _____

   B. List the stressors: _____

   _____

   _____

   _____

3. Enter city name: _____

   A. Stress ranking: _____

   B. List the stressors: _____

   _____

   _____

   _____

4. Enter city name: _____

   A. Stress ranking: _____

   B. List the stressors: _____

   _____

   _____

   _____

5. Enter your hometown: _____

   A. Stress ranking: _____

   B. List the stressors: _____

      _____

      _____

      _____

Question

1. How does your hometown compare to other cities on the list? Is it as stressful? less stressful? Explain your response.

_____

_____

_____

_____

_____

_____

_____

_____

_____

Lesson 6.1   Activity C

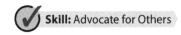

Stress Survey

Instructions: *Using the questions in this activity, survey five friends about their stressors. Record their responses as you administer the survey. Analyze these results and educate your classmates on common stressors and stress-management strategies.*

Friend 1

1. What is your stress level (from 1 to 5)? _____

2. What causes most of your stress?

   _____

3. How do you manage stress? Is this effective?

   _____

   _____

4. Whom do you feel you can go to for help?

   _____

Friend 2

1. What is your stress level (from 1 to 5)? _____

2. What causes most of your stress?

   _____

3. How do you manage stress? Is this effective?

   _____

   _____

4. Whom do you feel you can go to for help?

   _____

Friend 3

1. What is your stress level (from 1 to 5)? _____

2. What causes most of your stress?

   _____

3. How do you manage stress? Is this effective?

   _____

   _____

4. Whom do you feel you can go to for help?

   _____

Friend 4

1. What is your stress level (from 1 to 5)? _____

2. What causes most of your stress?

   _____

3. How do you manage stress? Is this effective?

   _____

   _____

4. Whom do you feel you can go to for help?

   _____

Friend 5

1. What is your stress level (from 1 to 5)? _____

2. What causes most of your stress?

   _____

3. How do you manage stress? Is this effective?

   _____

   _____

4. Whom do you feel you can go to for help?

   _____

Questions

1. Based on your data, are your friends feeling stressed? What are common stressors?

   _____

   _____

   _____

   _____

2. Based on your data, what effective strategies do your friends use to manage stress?

   _____

   _____

   _____

   _____

3. Share these stressors and stress management strategies with your class. Do your classmates experience similar stressors and use similar strategies? List any additional stressors or strategies mentioned.

   _____

   _____

   _____

   _____

   _____

Name _____ Date _____ Period _____

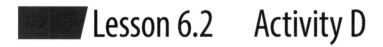 Lesson 6.2   Activity D

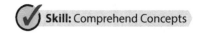

Physical Responses to Stress

Instructions: *For this activity, choose one stressful event that you and your friends have experienced. Record your physical response to this stressful event below. Then, ask at least two friends how their bodies responded to this stressful event. Record the responses and compare your results.*

1. Stressful event: _____
   _____

2. Your physical response: _____
   _____
   _____
   _____

3. Friend #1's physical response: _____
   _____
   _____
   _____

4. Friend #2's physical response: _____
   _____
   _____
   _____

5. How do your and your friends' physical responses compare? Do your bodies respond to stress in the same way, or were your responses quite different? Explain your answers.
   _____
   _____
   _____
   _____
   _____
   _____
   _____
   _____
   _____
   _____
   _____
   _____
   _____
   _____
   _____

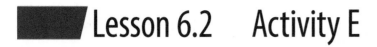 ## Lesson 6.2   Activity E

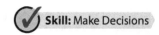

Mental Effects of Stress

Instructions: *Read the scenarios below and then identify the mental and emotional effects of stress each teen may be experiencing. Finally, describe decisions each teen can make to manage stress well.*

Scenario 1

Jaden and his family recently moved across town. While Jaden loves their new house, he now has to attend a different high school for his senior year. He wishes his parents would have waited until he had graduated to move. At his old school, Jaden was captain of the basketball team and had lots of friends. Jaden plans on joining the basketball team at his new school, but is worried this coach will not give him as much playing time as he had on his previous team. He's also finding it hard both to make new friends and spend time with his old friends.

1. What mental and emotional effects might stress have on Jaden?

_____

_____

2. What decision can Jaden make to manage this stress?

_____

Scenario 2

Maya is supposed to take the SAT on Friday. This will be her second time taking the test. The first time she took it, her score did not meet admissions requirements for the college she wants to attend. Maya hopes that by studying and taking practice exams, she will do much better this time. Unfortunately, it seems like every time she sits down to study, her younger brother and sister interrupt her.

1. What mental and emotional effects might stress have on Maya?

_____

_____

2. What decision can Maya make to manage this stress?

_____

Scenario 3

Dylan and Nivaan have been dating for most of their freshman year. Last week, Nivaan told Dylan she thinks they should just be friends. The two share a lot of friends, and Dylan is afraid Nivaan's friends will stop being friends with him now that he and Nivaan are no longer together. They are also in the same algebra, history, and French classes, and he worries those classes will be hard to sit through.

1. What mental and emotional effects might stress have on Dylan?

_____

_____

2. What decision can Dylan make to manage this stress?

_____

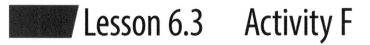 Lesson 6.3   Activity F   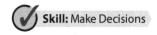 Skill: Make Decisions

How Would You Handle It?

Instructions: *For this activity, read the following scenarios and decide how you would handle the stress each individual is facing. Describe the pros and cons of your decision to explain why this is the healthiest decision.*

Scenario 1

Last month, Shana's parents announced they are getting a divorce. Shana was shocked—she had never even seen them fight! Since her dad moved out, Shana's mom has been crying a lot, and Shana feels guilty for going out with friends and leaving her mom alone.

1. How would you handle the stress Shana is facing? What are the pros and cons of this decision?

_____

_____

_____

_____

_____

_____

_____

_____

_____

_____

Scenario 2

Last month, Miguel's parents told him they cannot afford to help pay for college. In addition to school and multiple extracurricular activities, Miguel now works 15 hours each week at a part-time job. His grades are starting to slip and he's tired all the time.

1. How would you handle the stress Miguel is facing? What are the pros and cons of this decision?

_____

_____

_____

_____

_____

_____

_____

_____

_____

_____

Scenario 3

After Lyla's mom married her boyfriend, Dave, they moved into Dave's house. The house is twenty minutes from Lyla's hometown and she had to switch schools. Now, Lyla's mom and Dave have announced they're having a baby. Lyla feels left out and misses her old friends.

1. How would you handle the stress Lyla is facing? What are the pros and cons of this decision?

_____

_____

_____

_____

_____

_____

_____

_____

_____

_____

Scenario 4

Until last week when she broke her wrist at volleyball practice, Claire had been a starter on the team. Not being able to play has left Claire irritable, not to mention she feels like she has tons of energy to burn.

1. How would you handle the stress Claire is facing? What are the pros and cons of this decision?

_____

_____

_____

_____

_____

_____

_____

_____

_____

_____

Name _____ Date _____ Period _____

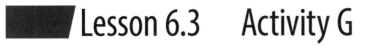 Lesson 6.3   Activity G   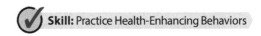 **Skill:** Practice Health-Enhancing Behaviors

Stress Management

Instructions: *Read the following scenarios. Identify the stressors in each person's life. Then, determine healthy stress management techniques the young people can use to cope with their stressors.*

1. Two months ago, Dax's grandfather died from cancer. Dax has never lost a close family member before and he feels disoriented. He misses his grandfather every day. He also worries about his mom and does what he can to cheer her up.

   A. Stressor(s): _____

   _____

   B. Healthy stress management techniques: _____

   _____

   _____

2. Ava dreads doing homework. She wants to do well, but everything she learns in class seems to fly from her brain when she leaves school. The more Ava stresses about it, the less she seems to remember and the more frustrated she becomes.

   A. Stressor(s): _____

   _____

   B. Healthy stress management techniques: _____

   _____

   _____

3. The forest fire that tore through Zion's home state last year came quickly. His parents barely had enough time to grab important documents before they were evacuated. By the time they returned to the area, Zion's childhood home was gone.

   A. Stressor(s): _____

   _____

   B. Healthy stress management techniques: _____

   _____

   _____

4. Riley has been physically abused for the last year by her boyfriend. She hides the bruises from her friends and family so they will not find out. Lately, the abuse has gotten more severe.

   A. Stressor(s): _____

   _____

   B. Healthy stress management techniques: _____

   _____

   _____

5. Every day, Chyna checks her phone to see meaner and angrier messages posted on her social media. When Chyna went to a teacher about it, the teacher said she did not have proof that it was other students sending these messages.

   A. Stressor(s): _____

   _____

   B. Healthy stress management techniques: _____

   _____

   _____

6. When Santiago gets off the bus and goes up to his door, he realizes that he left his keys in his locker at school. He pulls out his phone and sees that it has died. Santiago's dad will not be home for another few hours.

   A. Stressor(s): _____

   _____

   B. Healthy stress management techniques: _____

   _____

   _____

7. Aniya's single dad can no longer afford to pay rent for their apartment. They sleep in his car and Aniya's dad takes her to the local gym so she can shower each morning before school. Aniya worries that someone will find out and take her away from her dad.

   A. Stressor(s): _____

   _____

   B. Healthy stress management techniques: _____

   _____

   _____

8. Bella feels overwhelmed sometimes by social media. She loves that she can always talk to her friends, but the constant notifications make her feel like she needs to always be on her phone. Now and then, Bella just needs a break.

   A. Stressor(s): _____

   _____

   B. Healthy stress management techniques: _____

   _____

   _____

9. Finals at the end of the year are always really stressful for Austin. Each year, he worries that he will fail his tests and have to repeat a grade. This pressure makes it difficult for Austin to stay focused during his tests.

   A. Stressor(s): _____

   _____

   B. Healthy stress management techniques: _____

   _____

   _____

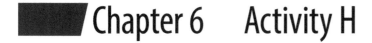 **Chapter 6   Activity H**

Practice Test

Completion

Instructions: *Write the term that completes the statement in the space provided.*

1. Repeated exposure to severe, chronic stressors can lead to _____ stress.

   _____

2. Your body's response to stress can be divided into three stages: alarm, _____, and exhaustion.

   _____

3. The body's _____ system defends against infection and disease.

   _____

4. A stress-related disorder people experience after an extremely frightening or upsetting event is _____.

   _____

5. Keeping a to-do list or avoiding procrastination are strategies for _____, a stress reduction practice.

   _____

True/False

Instructions: *Indicate whether each statement below is true or false.*

6. _____ *True or false?* School is the only source of stress for teens.

7. _____ *True or false?* Two people can experience the same stressor differently depending on their perceptions.

8. _____ *True or false?* Epinephrine, norepinephrine, and cortisol are known as the stress hormones.

9. _____ *True or false?* Stress does *not* affect a person's behaviors.

10. _____ *True or false?* Speaking to yourself in a way that reminds you of your positive qualities and your ability to cope with stress is positive reappraisal.

Multiple Choice

Instructions: *Select the letter that corresponds to the correct answer.*

11. _____ Which of the following is an example of eustress?
    A. conflict with your parents   C. losing your phone
    B. bullying at school   D. getting a driver's license

12. _____ The _____ system is responsible for prompting other body systems to react to stressful or threatening situations.
    A. immune   C. endocrine
    B. cardiovascular   D. nervous

13. _____ Stress affects _____, the ability to think, reason, and remember.
    A. perception   C. cognition
    B. visualization   D. deception

Matching

Instructions: *Match each key term to its definition (14–21).*

14. _____ act of thinking about the good aspects of stressful events

15. _____ relaxation technique that involves imagining one's self in a pleasant environment

16. _____ stress that causes negative feelings and harmful health effects

17. _____ relaxation technique that involves tensing and then relaxing each part of the body until the whole body feels relaxed

18. _____ body's physical and psychological reactions to situations people perceive as threats

19. _____ stress caused by repeated, long-lasting exposure to severe stressors

20. _____ state of emotional, physical, and mental exhaustion

21. _____ ability to think, reason, and remember

A. burnout
B. cognition
C. distress
D. positive reappraisal
E. progressive muscle relaxation
F. stress
G. toxic stress
H. visualization

Analyzing Data

Instructions: *The following chart presents data from the American Psychological Association about the stress management of teens. Use the information provided to answer the following questions.*

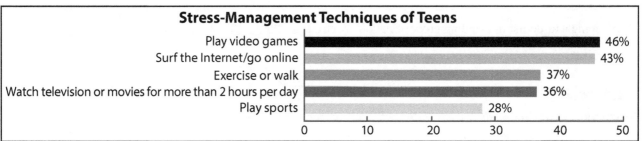

American Psychological Association

Figure 1. Percentage of stress-management techniques used by teens

22. Assuming 100 students responded to the survey, how many more students go online to relieve stress than play a sport?

_____

23. Are physically active strategies more or less helpful than technology use? Explain.

_____

_____

24. Identify two stress management techniques of teens *not* included in the chart.

_____

_____

Short Answer

Instructions: *Answer the following questions using what you have learned in this chapter.*

25. How might stress cause physical exhaustion?

_____

_____

26. Why is it wise to avoid using tobacco, alcohol, and drugs, particularly when experiencing stress?

_____

_____

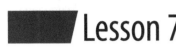

CHAPTER 7

Understanding Mental Illness

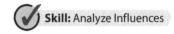

Lesson 7.1 Activity A

Skill: Analyze Influences

Which Factor?

Instructions: *Several factors contribute to the development of mental illnesses. Read each of the scenarios below and determine what factors may be an influence in each person's mental illness.*

1. Tim is a star on his high school football team. He plays in almost every game and has received awards for his performance. Playing football can be dangerous, though. After his most recent concussion, Tim acted strangely. He was anxious and even lashed out angrily at his friends when they offered their help.

   A. List factors of influence.

   _____

   _____

   _____

2. Recently, Malia's parents got divorced. At first, Malia thought she would be okay because her parents fight a lot. However, the stress of traveling between her mom's and dad's houses has started to affect her. She feels anxious at school, has trouble finishing assignments, and has obsessive-compulsive urges.

   A. List factors of influence.

   _____

   _____

   _____

3. Frankie is a straight-A student, but he often has low self-esteem. When he has trouble completing an assignment or does not get the right answer on his first try, Frankie's immediate thought is, "I'm a failure." No matter what his friends and family tell him, he cannot seem to shake the thought.

   A. List factors of influence.

   _____

   _____

   _____

4. For as long as Dana can remember, her mother has been very sad. Sometimes her mom would spend days in her bedroom and would not talk to anyone. Now, Dana realizes her mother has depression. Dana has begun to experience the same symptoms.

   A. List factors of influence.

   _____

   _____

   _____

Name _____ Date _____ Period _____

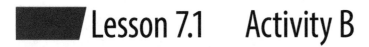

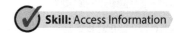

Identifying Mental Illnesses

Instructions: *In each of the following scenarios, the person described is experiencing a mental illness. Read each scenario and, using reliable resources, identify the possible mental illness described. Provide a citation for your research. Then, explain how that mental illness might affect the person's daily functioning.*

1. Mateo is at a concert with his friends. He was so excited to get tickets that he did not have time to think about the large crowd he would encounter. Halfway through the concert, Mateo begins to feel that something bad might happen. There are so many people in the concert hall, and the music seems to be getting louder. Mateo is nauseous and he can feel his heart racing.

    A. Possible mental illness: _____

    B. Reliable resource: _____

    C. Effects on daily functioning: _____

    _____

    _____

2. Mila's parents try to get her to organize her room, but she simply does not have enough space for all of her belongings. Mila knows that the issue is that she will throw nothing away—not old clothes that did not fit her, or magazines that she has finished reading, or a smartphone that no longer works. She has a gut feeling that if she throws any of these things away, something bad will happen. Keeping these items does not make that feeling go away, but she has to keep them.

    A. Possible mental illness: _____

    B. Reliable resource: _____

    C. Effects on daily functioning: _____

    _____

    _____

3. Corey, a freshman, is finding the transition to high school difficult. He cannot seem to pay attention in class, and he feels bored doing class assignments and activities. He forgets instructions the teacher gives, and often does assignments the wrong way as a result.

    A. Possible mental illness: _____

    B. Reliable resource: _____

    C. Effects on daily functioning: _____

    _____

    _____

4. Shannon just feels so tired. There is something about the cold weather and lack of sun in winter that makes her want to sleep until spring. When her uncle comes to her room to ask if she wants to cook with him like she loves to do, Shannon snaps, "Just leave me alone!" She has no idea why she is so cranky.

    A. Possible mental illness: _____

    B. Reliable resource: _____

    C. Effects on daily functioning: _____

    _____

    _____

Name _____ Date _____ Period _____

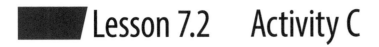 Lesson 7.2 Activity C

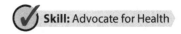

Mental Illness Treatment

Instructions: *Read the following scenarios about mental illnesses. Advocate for the health of others by helping Grace and Cody understand their treatment options. Explain how their friends can help support them, too. Do additional research as needed to complete this activity.*

Grace Cho (age 18)

Through initial conversations with a specialist, Grace learned that she needs professional treatment to manage her bipolar disorder. During her depressive episodes, Grace feels worthless and like she has no energy. When she feels manic, she does not sleep and feels like she cannot stop talking and moving. Grace is in need of a comprehensive approach to treatment.

1. What would you tell Grace about her need for treatment? What treatment options do you suggest? What might happen if Grace does not seek treatment?

_____

_____

_____

_____

_____

_____

2. What can Grace's friends do to help or support her?

_____

_____

Cody Green (age 13)

Cody excessively worries about being able to get through the day. He worries about waking up on time, driving safely to school, performing well in his classes, and maintaining relationships with his friends. Due to these worries, Cody has trouble sleeping and his body is sore from being so tense. He has a hard time concentrating on any tasks or conversations because of his constant worry.

1. What would you tell Cody about his need for treatment? What treatment options do you suggest? What might happen if Cody does not get treatment?

_____

_____

_____

_____

_____

_____

2. How can Cody's friends help or support him with his mental illness?

_____

_____

Name _____ Date _____ Period _____

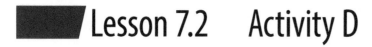 Lesson 7.2   Activity D

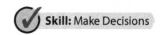

Choice and Outcomes

Instructions: *Read the following scenarios and imagine that you are the one with a mental illness. Identify the illness, indicate the pros and cons to getting help, and identify any possible barriers to getting help.*

Scenario 1

> You downloaded a game to your phone a few months ago. Your friends all played with you at first, but eventually they got bored and deleted the app. You play all day. The app is free to download, but at this point you have spent hundreds of dollars for upgrades and bonus items. That was all of your savings and birthday money, plus you told your parents you needed money for a nonexistent school trip. You cannot fall asleep at night without playing for a few hours and you now have trouble paying attention in class because you are thinking about the game.

1. What is the name of the mental illness? _____

2. What are the benefits to getting help?

   _____

   _____

3. What are some barriers to getting help?

   _____

   _____

4. Do you think the benefits outweigh the barriers? Explain.

   _____

   _____

Scenario 2

> The world does not make much sense to you anymore. Voices speak directly to you through the radio, which you know is not normal. A small child also seems to be following you around, but nobody else ever seems to see him. You are so distracted by these things that you have a hard time doing everyday tasks like going to school or taking a shower. Your mom says that you have started talking to yourself and she is worried about you. She has a lot to deal with as a single parent already.

1. What is the name of the mental illness? _____

2. What are the benefits to getting help?

   _____

   _____

3. What are some barriers to getting help?

   _____

   _____

4. Do you think the benefits outweigh the barriers? Explain.

   _____

   _____

Name _____ Date _____ Period _____

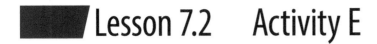 **Lesson 7.2   Activity E**

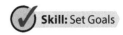

I Will Seek Help, If Needed

Instructions: *Seeking help for mental illnesses can be difficult. Fill out the following oath to yourself to help you seek help in the future if you need it.*

1. I will recognize I need help if I experience any of the following signs:

    A. Sign: _____

    B. Sign: _____

    C. Sign: _____

    D. Sign: _____

    E. Sign: _____

    F. Sign: _____

    G. Sign: _____

2. If I need help, I know the following resources are available in my community:

    A. Resource: _____

    B. Resource: _____

    C. Resource: _____

    D. Resource: _____

3. Therapy, medications, and inpatient treatment can all help me return to optimal health and are important services if I need them. Sometimes, however, the stigma around mental illnesses might stop me from seeking help. Here is one example of the stigma around mental illness and how I know it is untrue and unfair.

    A. Stigma: _____

    _____

    _____

    B. Reality: _____

    _____

    _____

4. I will remember that many people with negative beliefs about mental illnesses do not understand them. I will remember that I am not my mental illness. I will remember that my mental health is as important as my physical health.

    A. Signature: _____

Name _____ Date _____ Period _____

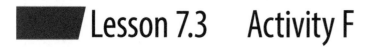 Lesson 7.3   Activity F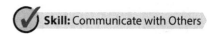

Suicide Prevention

Instructions: *In the following scenarios, identify any warning signs that are present. Then, write a short script for what you could say to show that you care, prevent a suicide attempt, and help them seek help.*

Scenario 1

> Your friend Aunika has been missing book club meetings. She used to love going to book club and often engaged in passionate discussions about the group's recent read. When you ask her about it, Aunika shrugs and says she hasn't been feeling up to attending the meetings. You find out from another friend of Aunika's that she has been missing her tennis lessons as well.

1. List the warning signs.

_____

_____

2. What would you say?

_____

_____

Scenario 2

> One day, your friend Caleb unexpectedly gives you his guitar. He saved up for two summers to buy that guitar and often said it was his most treasured possession. A few days later, your friend says that Caleb gave her a large portion of his book collection. Caleb just put the following message on social media: "If I killed myself, I bet no one would even miss me."

1. List the warning signs.

_____

_____

2. What would you say?

_____

_____

Scenario 3

> Michelle used to be your happiest, most upbeat friend. She was the chatterbox of your group, always ready to talk your ear off. Recently, however, Michelle has not been acting like herself. She has been broody and seems caught up in her own thoughts. When you asked her what was wrong, Michelle simply shrugged and continued scribbling in a notebook.

1. List the warning signs.

_____

_____

2. What would you say?

_____

_____

Name _____ Date _____ Period _____

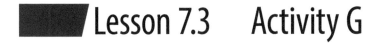 Lesson 7.3   Activity G

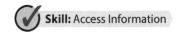

Mental Health Careers

Instructions: *When choosing a healthcare career, be mindful of your personal interests and qualities. These will help you decide which career would best suit you. Study the information in the chart below and answer the questions that follow. Do additional research as needed to complete the activity.*

Career	Interest/Quality	Duties	Education and Training	Resource
Psychiatrist	An interest in science Has good listening and communication skills	Diagnoses mental illnesses and disorders Must listen to patients and communicate treatments to them	Bachelor's degree, medical degree, certification exam	American Psychiatric Association
Psychiatric nurse	An interest in science Enjoys working with families	Tests patients to learn symptoms and patterns of illness Provides counseling to patients and their families	Nursing degree, specialized training in psychiatry and psychotherapy, direct clinical training	American Psychiatric Nurses Association
Psychologist	Enjoys working with people Has good listening and communication skills	Provides psychotherapy directly to patients Must listen to patients and communicate treatments to them	Doctoral degree, licensing exam	Society of Clinical Psychology
Clinical social worker	Enjoys working with people Has good listening and communication skills Enjoys a variety of workplaces	Treats patients directly for mental, behavioral, and emotional issues Must listen to patients and communicate treatments to them May work in mental health clinics, schools, hospitals, or private practice	Master's degree, supervised clinical therapy	National Association of Social Workers
Marriage and family therapist	Enjoys working with people and families Has good listening and communication skills Enjoys a variety of workplaces	Treats illnesses and disorders within families Must listen to couples and families and communicate treatments to them May work in a social work setting or in private practice	Bachelor's degree, sometimes a master's degree, direct clinical training	American Association for Marriage and Family Therapy

Figure 1. Information about mental health careers

1. Which of these careers most interests you? Explain why you think this career suits your interests and personal qualities.

_____

_____

_____

_____

_____

_____

2. Research this career further. Visit the resource listed in the chart for that career and compose a "day in the life" for someone with that career. Does this type of workday interest you?

_____

_____

_____

_____

_____

_____

3. According to the chart, what level of education is necessary for your chosen career?

_____

4. Research community colleges and universities in your area and plot out an educational plan to follow if you want this career.

_____

_____

_____

_____

_____

_____

_____

_____

_____

5. Visit the *Occupational Outlook Handbook* online to research the job outlook for this particular career. Record your findings here.

_____

_____

6. According to the *Occupational Outlook Handbook*, what is a typical salary for someone in this career?

_____

7. Based on your knowledge of this career, would you consider this career in the future? Why or why not?

_____

_____

_____

Name _____ Date _____ Period _____

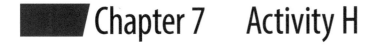 Chapter 7   Activity H

Practice Test

Completion

Instructions: *Write the term that completes the statement in the space provided.*

1. People with _____ disorder have recurring and uncontrollable thoughts, feelings, and behaviors that make daily functioning difficult.

   _____

2. An estimated 20 percent of people who are homeless may have a(n) _____ spectrum disorder.

   _____

3. The goal of _____ therapy is to help families build positive, functional relationships and strengthen interactions.

   _____

4. _____ medications slow down the central nervous system to help people feel calmer and more relaxed.

   _____

5. People with mental illnesses need _____ treatment if they are at serious risk of harming themselves or others.

   _____

True/False

Instructions: *Indicate whether each statement below is true or false.*

6. _____ *True or false?* The terms *mental illness* and *mental disorder* have different meanings.

7. _____ *True or false?* People with serious brain injuries are at a greater risk of developing a substance use disorder.

8. _____ *True or false?* A pregnant person's behaviors and experiences do *not* affect the mental health of the baby later in life.

9. _____ *True or false?* The most common reason people of any age attempt suicide is severe depression.

10. _____ *True or false?* People who experience long-term stress in their environments are more likely to attempt suicide.

Multiple Choice

Instructions: *Select the letter that corresponds to the correct answer.*

11. _____ Strong, unrealistic fear caused by an object or situation that does not really pose much danger is called a _____.
    A. social anxiety disorder   C. phobia
    B. mood disorder   D. conduct disorder

12. _____ People with _____ anxiety disorder feel extreme and constant anxiety about parts of their lives they cannot control.
    A. panic   C. social media
    B. social   D. generalized

13. _____ Which of the following is *not* a typical symptom of major depressive disorder?
    A. sudden, manic moods   C. extreme tiredness and loss of energy
    B. difficulty concentrating   D. recurrent thoughts of death

14. _____ Which of the following mental health medications make certain brain chemicals, such as serotonin, more available?
    A. antidepressants   C. mood stabilizers
    B. stimulants   D. antipsychotics

15. _____ A suicide _____ describes a series of suicides in a particular community over a relatively short period of time.
   A. clump
   B. cluster
   C. collection
   D. contagion

Matching

Instructions: *Match each key term to its definition (16–23).*

16. _____ health condition in which negative or unhelpful feelings or thoughts become so severe they interfere with daily life

17. _____ copying of suicide attempts after exposure to another person's suicide

18. _____ people who have lost someone to suicide

19. _____ negative, false, unfair beliefs associated with a circumstance, quality, or person

20. _____ mental illnesses characterized by irregular thoughts, delusions, and hallucinations

21. _____ mental illnesses in which feelings of worry and dread interfere with daily life

22. _____ two conditions that affect health at the same time

23. _____ treatment method that changes the way a person thinks, interprets information, behaves, and experiences and expresses emotions

A. anxiety disorders
B. co-occurring disorders
C. mental illness
D. schizophrenia spectrum disorder
E. stigma
F. suicide contagion
G. survivors
H. therapy

Analyzing Data

Instructions: *The chart below shows the rates of depressive symptoms, suicidal thoughts, and suicide attempts among female and male teens according to the US Department of Health and Human Services' Office of Adolescent Health. Study the data and answer the questions that follow.*

Depression and Suicide Among Students 12–17 Years of Age

Suicide Attempt — Female 10%, Male 6%
Suicidal Thoughts — Female 19%, Male 13%
Depressive Symptoms — Female 36%, Male 21%

US Department of Health and Human Services

Figure 2. Rates of depressive symptoms, suicidal thoughts, and suicide attempts among female and male teens

24. What percent more females than males experienced depressive symptoms?

_____

25. What percent of males and females did *not* attempt suicide?

_____

Short Answer

Instructions: *Answer the following questions using what you have learned in this chapter.*

26. What can you, as an individual, do to battle the social stigma surrounding mental illnesses?

_____

_____

27. What can you do to help a friend or loved one who is suffering from a mental illness?

_____

_____

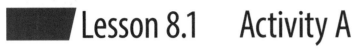

Following a Healthy Diet

Lesson 8.1 Activity A

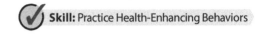
Skill: Practice Health-Enhancing Behaviors

Nutrient Review

Instructions: *Read the following scenarios and answer the questions about each person's nutrition.*

Scenario 1

Within the past three months, Janie has been to the doctor five times for a variety of illnesses. Today, Janie is back at the doctor's office with the flu. After examining her eating patterns, the doctor suggests eating healthier to strengthen her immune system.

1. Using the text for reference, list one vitamin and one mineral Janie should consume more of to strengthen her immune system. Then, list three foods that contain that vitamin and three that contain that mineral.

   A. Vitamin:_____

   Food source: _____

   Food source: _____

   Food source: _____

   B. Mineral:_____

   Food source: _____

   Food source: _____

   Food source: _____

Scenario 2

Carl, age 45, has recently been diagnosed with high cholesterol. His doctor tells him that he has to limit a certain type of fat to prevent long-term health conditions. He knows, however, that it is still important to eat some fats in his diet.

1. What type of fat is associated with elevated levels of cholesterol in the blood?

   _____

2. List three health conditions Carl is at risk for if he continues eating patterns high in this type of fat.

   _____

   _____

   _____

3. Provide three examples of healthy fats Carl can include in his diet.

   _____

   _____

   _____

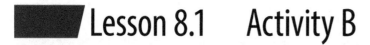 Lesson 8.1   Activity B

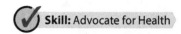

You Are the Chef

Instructions: *Design a nutrient-filled day for your family. Each meal must contain at least six vitamins and six minerals. Include beverages in your meal plan. Identify the vitamins and minerals contained in the food.*

What Is for Breakfast?

1. List the food and beverage items in this meal.

_____

2. List six vitamins contained in this meal.

_____

3. List six minerals contained in this meal.

_____

What Is for Lunch?

1. List the food and beverage items in this meal.

_____

2. List six vitamins contained in this meal.

_____

3. List six minerals contained in this meal.

_____

What Is for Dinner?

1. List the food and beverage items in this meal.

_____

2. List six vitamins contained in this meal.

_____

3. List six minerals contained in this meal.

_____

Question

1. Describe how these meals would benefit your family's bodies. Be specific and provide at least five examples.

_____

_____

_____

_____

_____

Name _____ Date _____ Period _____

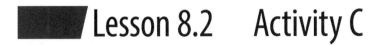 Lesson 8.2   Activity C

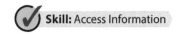

Evaluate Your Diet

Instructions: *In this four-part activity, compare what you are eating now to what the Dietary Guidelines for Americans recommends.*

Part 1: Complete a Three-Day Food Log

Instructions: *Record everything you eat and drink for three days. This includes meals, snacks, and water and other beverages. Estimate the serving size for every food or beverage you consume.*

1. Day 1: What did you eat and drink?

_____

_____

_____

2. Day 2: What did you eat and drink?

_____

_____

_____

3. Day 3: What did you eat and drink?

_____

_____

_____

Part 2: Sort Foods into Food Groups

Instructions: *Review your food log from the past three days, and assign each item in your log to one or more food groups.*

1. Grains

   A. Day 1: _____   C. Day 3: _____

   B. Day 2: _____   D. Total servings: _____

2. Protein foods

   A. Day 1: _____   C. Day 3: _____

   B. Day 2: _____   D. Total servings: _____

3. Fruits

   A. Day 1: _____   C. Day 3: _____

   B. Day 2: _____   D. Total servings: _____

4. Vegetables

   A. Day 1: _____   C. Day 3: _____

   B. Day 2: _____   D. Total servings: _____

5. Dairy

    A. Day 1: _____

    B. Day 2: _____

6. Added sugars

    A. Day 1: _____

    B. Day 2: _____

    C. Day 3: _____

    D. Total servings: _____

    C. Day 3: _____

    D. Total servings: _____

Part 3: Research Recommended Amounts

Instructions: *For each food group, calculate the average number of servings you ate each day for each food group. Research the amount of each food group recommended for you based on your age, biological sex, height, weight, and level of physical activity. Then, calculate the difference between your current eating pattern and the recommended one.*

1. Grains

    A. Average amount over three days: _____

    B. Recommended amount: _____

    C. Difference: _____

2. Protein foods

    A. Average amount over three days: _____

    B. Recommended amount: _____

    C. Difference: _____

3. Fruits

    A. Average amount over three days: _____

    B. Recommended amount: _____

    C. Difference: _____

4. Vegetables

    A. Average amount over three days: _____

    B. Recommended amount: _____

    C. Difference: _____

5. Dairy

    A. Average amount over three days: _____

    B. Recommended amount: _____

    C. Difference: _____

6. Added sugars

    A. Average amount over three days: _____

    B. Recommended amount: _____

    C. Difference: _____

Part 4: Drawing Conclusions

Instructions: *Review the results of your calculations from Part 3, and then answer the following questions.*

1. Did you eat more than the recommended amount in any food group? Which group(s)?

_____

_____

2. Did you eat less than the recommended amount in any food group? Which group(s)?

_____

_____

3. Based on your three-day food log, what changes, if any, would you make to eat healthier? Be specific.

_____

_____

_____

_____

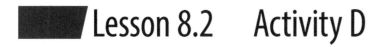 Lesson 8.2   Activity D

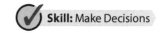 **Skill:** Make Decisions

Evaluating Nutrient Density

Instructions: *Using an online nutrient database, fill in the information below with how many calories are contained in each meal and which nutrients are provided by each food such as carbohydrates, protein, fats, vitamins, and minerals. Then answer the questions that follow.*

Meal Options

1. **Fried chicken and fries:** 3 drumsticks deep-fried chicken, medium serving French fries

   A. Total calories: _____

   B. Nutrients supplied: _____

   _____

2. **Turkey wrap:** 1 whole-wheat tortilla, 2 slices turkey breast, 1/4 c. raw bell peppers and onions, 2 tsp. fat-free mustard

   A. Total calories: _____

   B. Nutrients supplied: _____

   _____

3. **Grilled chicken salad:** 2 c. lettuce, 3 oz. skinless grilled chicken breast, 1/2 c. bread croutons, 1 Tbsp. low-fat mayo

   A. Total calories: _____

   B. Nutrients supplied: _____

   _____

4. **Chicken and veggie bowl:** 4 oz. skinless grilled chicken breast, 1 c. roasted sweet potatoes, 1 c. spinach and green beans, 2 Tbsp. brown mustard

   A. Total calories: _____

   B. Nutrients supplied: _____

   _____

Questions

5. Describe the pros and cons of each meal option.

   A. Fried chicken and fries: _____

   _____

   _____

   _____

   B. Turkey wrap: _____

   _____

   _____

   _____

C. Grilled chicken salad: _____

_____

_____

_____

D. Chicken and veggie bowl: _____

_____

_____

_____

6. Identify the best meal option. Support your choice with information about nutrients.

_____

_____

_____

7. Finally, create your own healthy option with your favorite nutrient-dense foods. List four food items and the nutrients provided.

A. Food item: _____

Nutrients provided: _____

_____

B. Food item: _____

Nutrients provided: _____

_____

C. Food item: _____

Nutrients provided: _____

_____

D. Food item: _____

Nutrients provided: _____

_____

Name _____ Date _____ Period _____

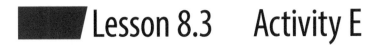 Lesson 8.3   Activity E

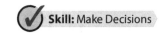

Decision-Making at the Grocery Store

Instructions: *Luke goes grocery shopping for his family. He wants to fill his cart with the most nutritious items for his family. Review each set of alternatives and decide which product Luke should add to his cart.*

1. Decide which product Luke should add to his cart. Explain your answer.
    A. **Product A:** Ground beef, 1 lb. 51 grams saturated fat
    B. **Product B:** Ground turkey, 1 lb. 12.2 grams saturated fat

    _____

    _____

    _____

2. Decide which product Luke should add to his cart. Explain your answer.
    A. **Product A:** Whole-grain bread; **Ingredients:** 100% whole grain whole wheat flour, wheat fiber, water, wheat gluten, yeast, brown sugar
    B. **Product B:** White bread; **Ingredients:** Enriched bleached flour, water, high fructose corn syrup, yeast

    _____

    _____

    _____

3. Decide which product Luke should add to his cart. Explain your answer.
    A. **Product A:** Mint chocolate chip ice cream; 300 calories per serving (1 cup)
    B. **Product B:** Chocolate fudge brownie ice cream; 150 calories per serving (1/3 cup)

    _____

    _____

    _____

4. Decide which product Luke should add to his cart. Explain your answer.
    A. **Product A:** Peanut butter chocolate protein bar; 220 calories, 12 grams fat, 10 grams protein, 8 grams added sugar
    B. **Product B:** Blueberry protein bar; 210 calories, 7 grams fat, 12 grams protein, 0 grams added sugar

    _____

    _____

    _____

5. Decide which product Luke should add to his cart. Explain your answer.
    A. **Product A:** Grape juice; **Ingredients:** Sugar, water, natural and artificial flavors, citric acid, tartaric acid, grape juice, sucralose
    B. **Product B:** Apple juice; **Ingredients:** Filtered water, apple juice from concentrate, natural flavors, vitamin C, citric acid

    _____

    _____

    _____

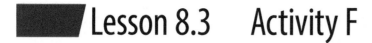 **Lesson 8.3   Activity F**

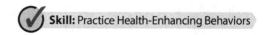

Practicing Food-Safety Behaviors

Instructions: *Read each of the following scenarios and identify the food-safety hazards. Explain what each person can do to practice better food safety.*

Scenario 1

Xavier decided this morning he wanted to grill chicken. He took his chicken out of the freezer, unwrapped it, and set it on the counter to thaw throughout the day. Then, he cuts pieces of the raw chicken on a cutting board. He seasons the chicken and puts the pieces on the grill. While the chicken is cooking, Xavier makes a salad using the same cutting board to chop the vegetables. Because he is in a hurry, Xavier does not wash his hands.

1. List two food-safety hazards in this scenario.

_____

2. What should Xavier do differently?

_____

_____

Scenario 2

One night, Amanda postpones cleaning up after dinner to go to a movie with friends. Four hours later, Amanda returns to the kitchen where the uneaten food is still in serving dishes on the counter. She covers the dishes and puts the food into the refrigerator so she and her family can eat the leftovers. She then wipes up the counters and table with a dry paper towel and washes the dishes in cold water with no soap.

1. List two food-safety hazards in this scenario.

_____

2. What should Amanda do differently?

_____

_____

Scenario 3

Jamila makes a veggie tray with a yogurt-based dip as a snack for herself. She prepares the bell peppers, broccoli, and snap peas and puts them on a plate. They did not seem dirty, so Jamila does not wash them. She goes to sit outside because the weather is so nice and warm. Her friend stops by a few hours later and Jamila offers her some veggies and yogurt dip.

1. List two food-safety hazards in this scenario.

_____

2. What should Jamila do differently?

_____

_____

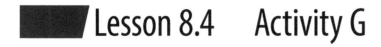 Lesson 8.4   Activity G

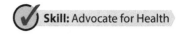 **Skill:** Advocate for Health

Danger with Comparisons

Instructions: *Read the following situations where a teen might feel self-conscious about their body. Explain how this comparison may not give each teen an accurate look at their weight.*

1. Kiera and Mary are both 14 and still growing. They are currently the same height, but Kiera weighs 15 more pounds than Mary.

   A. Describe the danger with comparisons.

   _____

   _____

   _____

2. Janet finds out that her body-fat percentage is 25%. Her boyfriend, Darius, has a body-fat percentage of 15%.

   A. Describe the danger with comparisons.

   _____

   _____

   _____

3. At 14 years old, Trevor is 5 feet 9 inches tall, and wishes he looked more like his family friend, Louis. Louis is 17, and even though he weighs about the same as Trevor, Louis is 6 feet tall.

   A. Describe the danger with comparisons.

   _____

   _____

   _____

4. In middle school, Kris and Nancy often shared and swapped clothes. By tenth grade, however, Kris can no longer fit into Nancy's clothing because her hips have grown wider.

   A. Describe the danger with comparisons.

   _____

   _____

   _____

5. Lawrence and Diego, both 17 years old, are cousins. Diego is a member of the swim team and exercises regularly. Lawrence does not work out, and yet weighs 20 pounds less than Diego.

   A. Describe the danger with comparisons.

   _____

   _____

   _____

Instructions: *In small groups, create a campaign to inform students at your school about the drawbacks of comparing their bodies to other people's.*

Name _____ Date _____ Period _____

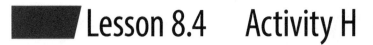 Lesson 8.4   Activity H

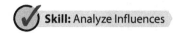

Identifying Unhealthy Eating Factors

Instructions: *For each of the following scenarios, identify the factors that impact each person's weight.*

Scenario 1

> Several times a week, Serena's family meets for big potluck meals. Using large serving spoons, they scoop food onto their plates from the serving dishes piled high with delicious foods. Many of Serena's family members, including her parents, are affected by overweight and obesity. Recently, Serena's doctor has told her she is in the overweight category.

1. What factors may be influencing Serena's weight?

   _____

   _____

2. What can Serena do to manage her weight?

   _____

   _____

Scenario 2

> When he is angry, sad, or anxious, Julio reaches for his favorite junk foods. Eating ice cream, pizza rolls, or popcorn makes him feel better. However, his emotions return when he finishes his snack. Julio has noticed that he has extra fat that his body stores mostly in his abdomen.

1. What factors may be influencing Julio's weight?

   _____

   _____

2. What can Julio do to manage his weight?

   _____

   _____

Scenario 3

> Since he stays up late most nights, Chris wakes up tired and with no time to eat breakfast. Instead, he will grab an energy drink on his way out the door. Wrestling practices often keep him busy during dinnertime, so he often skips that meal altogether. His coach recently pulled him aside and expressed his concern that Chris' weight is below the typical range for boys his age and height.

1. What factors may be influencing Chris' weight?

   _____

   _____

2. What can Chris do to manage his weight?

   _____

   _____

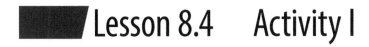 Lesson 8.4   Activity I

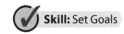

Weight-Management Goal Setting

Instructions: *Read the following scenario and help Jeremy set a goal to lose weight safely.*

Jeremy, who is 16 years old, spends much of his free time watching TV or texting his friends. He used to play hockey and soccer, but since his best friend moved away, he quit those activities. Most days he stops by a fast-food restaurant where he orders a milkshake for an after-school snack. He stays up late doing homework and watching TV, so he does not get enough sleep. For the past four years, Jeremy's weight has been slowly climbing. At his last physical examination, his doctor explained that he is 15 pounds above the healthy weight range for male teens his age and height. His doctor recommended that Jeremy lose the weight before he develops any health conditions.

1. First, help Jeremy assess the situation by answering the following questions.

   A. Why is Jeremy's weight gain a concern?

   _____

   _____

   B. What factors have influenced this weight gain?

   _____

   _____

   C. Why does Jeremy need to do something about it now?

   _____

   _____

2. Write a central goal that will help Jeremy lose 15 pounds within 10 weeks. (**Reminder:** Effective, gradual weight loss keeps a pace of 1–2 pounds per week.)

   _____

   _____

3. To be sure your goal is SMART, indicate how it meets each of the following.

   A. Specific: _____

   B. Measurable: _____

   C. Achievable: _____

   D. Relevant: _____

   E. Timely: _____

4. Define the steps Jeremy can take to achieve this goal.

   A. How can Jeremy break down his goal into smaller, more manageable steps that fit his 10-week time frame?

   _____

   _____

   _____

   _____

   _____

   B. List actions Jeremy can take to burn more calories.

   _____

   _____

C. List actions Jeremy can take to consume fewer calories.

_____

_____

5. While it is great that Jeremy has a goal, he must enact his plan. Describe some support systems and resources Jeremy can put in place to make acting on his goal more likely.

_____

_____

_____

6. Create a brief checklist for Jeremy to measure how he is progressing.

A. _____ Item: _____

B. _____ Item: _____

C. _____ Item: _____

D. _____ Item: _____

E. _____ Item: _____

F. _____ Item: _____

G. _____ Item: _____

H. _____ Item: _____

I. _____ Item: _____

J. _____ Item: _____

7. Self-rewards will help Jeremy keep himself motivated to achieve his goal. What reward could Jeremy put in place for himself

A. after his first week?

_____

B. halfway through his time line?

_____

C. when he achieves his goal?

_____

■■■ Chapter 8   Activity J

Practice Test

Completion

Instructions: *Write the term that completes the statement in the space provided.*

1. The body uses _____ to build and maintain muscles, bones, skin, hair, nails, and other organs.

   _____

2. Through digestion, the carbohydrates you eat are broken down to become _____, the body's preferred source of energy.

   _____

3. A(n) _____ food is rich in vitamins and minerals and has little to no saturated fats, added sugars, or sodium.

   _____

4. Substances added to food products to cause desired changes, such as to flavor or shelf life, are called food _____.

   _____

5. Waist circumference and waist-to-hip ratio are methods used to assess _____ distribution.

   _____

True/False

Instructions: *Indicate whether each statement below is true or false.*

6. _____ *True or false?* People should avoid eating any fats, if possible.

7. _____ *True or false?* Consuming more of some nutrients, such as added sugars, saturated fats, sodium, or refined grains, than a person needs can lead to overnutrition.

8. _____ *True or false?* In a food label's ingredients list, ingredients are listed by how nutritious they are.

9. _____ *True or false?* Females have a higher percentage of body fat than males.

10. _____ *True or false?* Muscle and bone weigh less than fat.

Multiple Choice

Instructions: *Select the letter that corresponds to the correct answer.*

11. _____ Your body requires only very small amounts of _____ to function properly.
    A. carbohydrates   C. proteins
    B. water   D. vitamins

12. _____ _____ is a complex carbohydrate that the body cannot completely break down.
    A. Dietary fiber   C. Fructose
    B. *Trans* fat   D. Protein

13. _____ The energy provided by food is measured in a unit called a _____.
    A. pound   C. degree
    B. calorie   D. gram

14. _____ _____ is a food guidance system that reminds people about the proportions of each food group they should eat at a meal.
    A. The *Dietary Guidelines for Americans*   C. A Nutrition Facts label
    B. Daily Values   D. MyPlate

15. _____ The rates of _____ doubled for adults and tripled for children from 1980–2008.
   A. overweight   C. healthy weight
   B. underweight   D. obesity

Matching

Instructions: *Match each key term to its definition (16–22).*

16. _____ stylish weight-loss plans that promise significant weight loss in short periods of time, often through cutting out food groups or buying premade meals

17. _____ produced without the use of chemical fertilizers, pesticides, or other artificial chemicals

18. _____ substances that help the body eliminate sodium and water, mostly through increased urination

19. _____ rate at which the body uses energy to carry out basic physiological processes

20. _____ inorganic nutrients absorbed from plants, water, and animal food sources

21. _____ tool used to determine whether a person's weight is healthy for that person's height

22. _____ ratio of the various components—fat, bone, and muscle—that make up the body

A. body composition
B. body mass index
C. diuretics
D. fad diets
E. metabolism
F. minerals
G. organic

Analyzing Data

Instructions: *Use the Nutrition Facts labels provided to answer the following questions.*

23. If someone eats three servings of Food B, how many grams of added sugars would this person consume?

   _____

   _____

24. If a person on a 2,000-calorie eating plan eats 1.5 cups of Food A, what percent of the Daily Value for sodium would this be?

   _____

   _____

25. Which food contains the most calcium per serving?

   _____

   _____

Food A

Nutrition Facts
17 servings per container
Serving size   3/4 cup (28g)

Amount per serving
Calories   110

	% Daily Value*
Total Fat 1.5g	2%
Saturated Fat 0g	0%
Trans Fat 0g	
Cholesterol 0mg	0%
Sodium 160mg	7%
Total Carbohydrate 22g	4%
Dietary Fiber 2g	7%
Total Sugars 9g	
Includes 8g Added Sugars	16%
Protein 2g	

Vitamin D 1mcg 5%	Calcium 104mg 8%
Iron 4.5mg 25%	Potassium 115mg 2%

* The % Daily Value (DV) tells you how much a nutrient in a serving of food contributes to a daily diet. 2,000 calories a day is used for general nutrition advice.

Food B

Nutrition Facts
1 serving per container
Serving size   1 cup (245g)

Amount per serving
Calories   208

	% Daily Value*
Total Fat 3g	4%
Saturated Fat 2g	10%
Trans Fat 0g	
Cholesterol 12mg	4%
Sodium 162mg	7%
Total Carbohydrate 34g	12%
Dietary Fiber 0g	0%
Total Sugars 34g	
Includes 17g Added Sugars	34%
Protein 12g	

Vitamin D 0mcg	0%
Calcium 419mg	32%
Iron 0.2mg	1%
Potassium 537mg	11%

* The % Daily Value (DV) tells you how much a nutrient in a serving of food contributes to a daily diet. 2,000 calories a day is used for general nutrition advice.

Figure 1. Nutrition Facts labels

Short Answer

Instructions: *Answer the following questions using what you have learned in this chapter.*

26. Explain the concept of maintaining calorie balance. What happens when calorie balance is *not* maintained?

   _____

   _____

27. Give an example of an "all-or-nothing" mind-set about eating, and explain how it can undermine weight-management efforts.

   _____

   _____

CHAPTER 9 — Having a Healthy Body Image

Lesson 9.1   Activity A

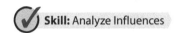
Skill: Analyze Influences

Media Messages About Body Types

Instructions: *Many types of media idealize a particular shape and size of male and female bodies. In this activity, find and analyze the messages about body type given in one advertisement and one TV program.*

Advertisement

1. Where did you find this advertisement?

   _____

2. What product or service is the advertisement selling?

   _____

3. Who is the target audience of this advertisement?

   _____

4. How does this advertisement portray an idealized body type?

   _____

   _____

5. What influence does this portrayal have on the target audience?

   _____

   _____

   _____

TV Program

1. What is the name of the TV program?

   _____

2. Who is the target audience of this program?

   _____

3. How does this program portray an idealized body type?

   _____

   _____

4. What influence does this portrayal have on the target audience?

   _____

   _____

   _____

Name _____ Date _____ Period _____

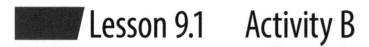
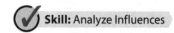
What Impacts My Body Image?

Instructions: *Read the following scenarios and answer the questions about the influences that can affect a teen's body image.*

Scenario 1

At 15 years old, Mlo is the shortest guy in his family. He feels self-conscious about his height every day. Mlo's family teases him about his height, calling him "short stuff" and "nugget." People at school have not mentioned his height, and other guys are around the same height, but Mlo worries they make fun of him behind his back. A girl Mlo likes asked him to a school dance, and he said "no" because she is taller than him and he was embarrassed.

1. What factor influences Mlo's body image? Explain.

_____

_____

2. How does this factor disrupt Mlo's daily interactions?

_____

Scenario 2

For Naomi's ethnicity, curves symbolize feminine beauty in a way that she fears is not achievable for her. At 16, Naomi is still mostly flat-chested and has a similar lack of curves elsewhere. Her mom reassures her that girls grow at different rates, and that she is just "a late bloomer." Naomi worries, however, that she just has a thin, straight body that male members of her ethnicity might not find attractive.

1. What factor influences Naomi's body image? Explain.

_____

_____

2. Do you think that people in any ethnicity can find beauty in all shapes and sizes of bodies? Explain your answer.

_____

Scenario 3

Wyatt has loved playing basketball for as long as he can remember. This year, Wyatt made the varsity team at his high school. Since then, Wyatt has become uncomfortable with how his body compares to his older teammates and their opponents. They all seem so much more muscular than him. They look more like his favorite professional basketball players. Wyatt feels skinny and weak in relation. He worries like he looks like a little kid out on the court during games.

1. What factor influences Wyatt's body image? Explain.

_____

_____

2. How can Wyatt get physical activity and feel good about his body?

_____

Name _____ Date _____ Period _____

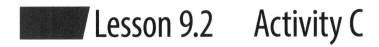 ## Lesson 9.2 Activity C

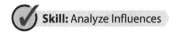 **Skill:** Analyze Influences

What Causes Disordered Eating?

Instructions: *Evaluate each of the following scenarios and identify factors that you think influence each teen to have disordered eating behaviors.*

Scenario 1

Fifteen-year-old Denise has been in gymnastics since she was a young girl. Her dream is to make the national team. Denise believes that she must stay small and thin to beat out her competitors. She does not see flaws in the bodies of anyone she competes against, and Denise feels like she needs to try harder to look like them. Although she has a healthy weight for her size, she engages in disordered eating behaviors to become even thinner.

1. Which factors influence Denise's disordered eating behaviors? Explain.

_____

_____

_____

_____

Scenario 2

Michael's friends call him the "human vacuum cleaner" because of the massive amounts of food he consumes in one sitting. Michael does not like the teasing, but eating this way calms him down temporarily when he feels anxious—which is often. He does not enjoy eating when he is already full, but Michael does not know how else to cope with his anxiety.

1. Which factors influence Michael's disordered eating behaviors? Explain.

_____

_____

_____

_____

Scenario 3

Juliana looks like any other healthy, active 16-year-old. However, she has disordered eating behaviors that no one knows about. Juliana does not have close friends who might notice these behaviors because she was bullied about her weight at school and is now afraid of trying to make new friends. At home, Juliana's parents are not usually around during dinnertime. She feels like no one notices because no one cares.

1. Which factors influence Juliana's disordered eating behaviors? Explain.

_____

_____

_____

_____

Name _____ Date _____ Period _____

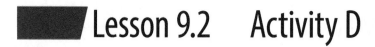 Lesson 9.2   Activity D

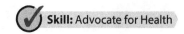 Skill: Advocate for Health

Battling Disordered Eating

Instructions: *List health conditions associated with disordered eating and eating disorders. Then, answer the following questions.*

Health Conditions Associated with Disordered Eating

1. Cardiovascular conditions: _____

_____

_____

2. Digestive conditions: _____

_____

_____

3. Nervous conditions: _____

_____

_____

4. Endocrine conditions: _____

_____

_____

5. Other conditions: _____

_____

_____

Questions

1. What mental and social effects might disordered eating behaviors or eating disorders have on a person?

_____

_____

_____

2. What professional organization can people contact if they need help making a plan and finding treatment for eating disorders? How can someone contact this organization on the phone, online, and by text?

_____

_____

_____

3. List three things that therapy can achieve for people with eating disorders.

_____

_____

_____

Name _____ Date _____ Period _____

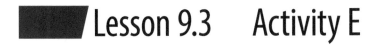 **Lesson 9.3   Activity E**

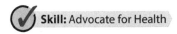

The Impact of Government

Instructions: *Review the section on advocating for positive body image in the text. Reflect on the efforts of other countries to promote the use of healthier body images in the media. Write a letter to US lawmakers to encourage legislation that promotes healthier body images. Use the guide below to outline your message.*

1. Who is a US lawmaker you believe can make a difference in the legislation that might affect body image? Explain.

_____

_____

_____

2. How can you contact this person?

_____

_____

3. What benefits can positive body image laws have on the general population?

_____

_____

_____

_____

4. What benefits can positive body image laws have on impressionable teens?

_____

_____

_____

_____

5. What strategies do you think can make a positive impact on the body image of teens? List at least three.

_____

_____

_____

_____

_____

_____

_____

_____

_____

Instructions: *Write your letter to this person using the benefits and strategies outlined above. Make sure to be clear, use appropriate language, and thank the person for their time. Send this letter to the person.*

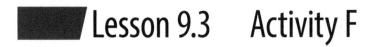 ## Lesson 9.3   Activity F

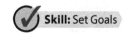

Building Up Your Body Image

Instructions: *Answer the following questions to develop a SMART goal to improve your body image. Keep in mind the strategies laid out in Lesson 9.3: viewing media critically, valuing your whole self, acknowledging diversity, checking your self-talk, avoiding negative influences, and advocating for positive body image.*

1. In what areas would you like to see improvement in your body image?

   _____

   _____

   _____

2. Create a central goal to achieve this objective.

   _____

   _____

   _____

3. To be sure your goal is SMART, indicate how it meets each of the following.

   A. Specific: _____

   B. Measurable: _____

   C. Achievable: _____

   D. Relevant: _____

   E. Timely: _____

4. List three short-term goals that will help you achieve your larger goal.

   A. Goal: _____

   _____

   B. Goal: _____

   _____

   C. Goal: _____

   _____

5. Name one obstacle that might stop you from achieving your goal. How can you overcome this obstacle?

   _____

   _____

   _____

   _____

   _____

   _____

6. Whom can you reach out to for help or support in going after your goal?

   _____

   _____

Name _____ Date _____ Period _____

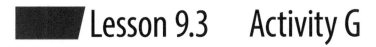 Lesson 9.3   Activity G   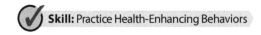 **Skill:** Practice Health-Enhancing Behaviors

Improving Your Body Image

Instructions: *Many people, teens included, spend much time focusing on what they dislike about their bodies. This negatively affects their body image. In this activity, reflect on positive things about your body and yourself. If you have difficulty completing the lists, ask a good friend or family member for input.*

1. List at least five things your body enables you to do.

   _____

   _____

   _____

   _____

   _____

2. List three metabolic activities that your body carries out to keep you alive. (For example, breathing.)

   _____

   _____

   _____

3. List ten things you like about yourself, including your physical appearance and your personal character traits.

   _____

   _____

   _____

   _____

   _____

   _____

   _____

   _____

   _____

   _____

4. Explain how your body is unique to you. Describe how, despite what is typically shown in the media, people appreciate many different body shapes, sizes, and looks.

   _____

   _____

   _____

   _____

   _____

   _____

   _____

   _____

5. Write three statements about your body that demonstrate positive self-talk.

_____

_____

_____

_____

_____

_____

_____

_____

_____

_____

Instructions: *Imagine that you have been chosen to be featured as a company's ambassador on social media. The company will post three images with captions that will highlight your shining qualities. Use the lists you collected (1–5). Write the captions about yourself for this company to use.*

1. Caption #1: _____

_____

2. Caption #2: _____

_____

3. Caption #3: _____

_____

Chapter 9   Activity H

Practice Test

Completion

Instructions: *Write the term that completes the statement in the space provided.*

1. A process that digitally alters an image to eliminate blemishes, cellulite, bulges, or wrinkles is _____.

   _____

2. The relationships in your life and the community around you, known as your _____ environment, influence your body image.

   _____

3. A disordered eating pattern called _____ is characterized by an obsession with healthy eating that leads to negative health consequences.

   _____

4. Fine hair that grows all over the body as a result of starvation is called _____.

   _____

5. Body _____ helps you focus on what bodies can do instead of how they look.

   _____

True/False

Instructions: *Indicate whether each statement below is true or false.*

6. _____ *True or false?* Your body image is determined by what your body actually looks like.

7. _____ *True or false?* The preference for a thin body type for females in the media is relatively new.

8. _____ *True or false?* Most teens do *not* feel self-conscious about their bodies.

9. _____ *True or false?* Eating disorders frequently go away on their own as people grow.

10. _____ *True or false?* Societal and family expectations are risk factors for disordered eating and eating disorders.

Multiple Choice

Instructions: *Select the letter that corresponds to the correct answer.*

11. _____ Factors that can influence a person's body image include _____.
    A family and peers
    B. images in the media
    C participation in athletic activities
    D All of the above.

12. _____ Which athletic activity emphasizes thin body types?
    A basketball
    B. soccer
    C softball
    D gymnastics

13. _____ Which of the following is a mental and emotional warning sign of an eating disorder?
    A feeling cold all the time
    B. frequent dieting
    C discomfort eating around others
    D withdrawal from friends and family

14. _____ Which of the following means accepting, caring, and being kind toward one's body?
    A body neutrality
    B. body positivity
    C body compassion
    D body empathy

Matching

Instructions: *Match each key term to its definition (15–22).*

15. _____ disorder characterized by extreme concern with becoming more muscular

16. _____ feelings of acceptance, care, and kindness toward one's body

17. _____ appreciation of body-type diversity

18. _____ focus on what the body can do, rather than how it looks

19. _____ range of irregular eating behaviors

20. _____ disordered eating pattern characterized by an obsession with healthy eating

21. _____ infrequent or delayed hard, dry bowel movements

22. _____ mental illness characterized by abnormal eating or disturbances in eating habits

A body compassion
B. body neutrality
C body positivity
D. constipation
E disordered eating
F. eating disorder
G muscle dysmorphia
H orthorexia

Analyzing Data

Instructions: *The table below presents data from the National Eating Disorder Association (NEDA). Use the data given to answer the questions that follow.*

Category	Trying to Lose Weight	Actively Dieting	Exercising to Lose Weight or Avoid Gaining Weight
Teen females	62.3%	58.6%	68.4%
Teen males	28.8%	28.2%	51.0%

National Eating Disorder Association (NEDA)

Figure 1. The National Center on Addiction and Substance Abuse (CASA) at Columbia University. Food for Thought: Substance Abuse and Eating Disorders.

23. If 2,500 teen males participated in this survey, how many would be exercising with the goal of losing weight or avoiding weight gain?

_____

_____

24. According to this study, what percentage of teen females are *not* attempting to lose weight?

_____

Short Answer

Instructions: *Answer the following questions using what you have learned in this chapter.*

25. Does happiness hinge on how a person looks? Explain your answer.

_____

_____

_____

26. Should extremely thin models be banned from fashion shows, advertisements, and publications in the US? Explain your answer.

_____

_____

_____

_____

_____

CHAPTER 10 Engaging in Physical Activity

Lesson 10.1   Activity A   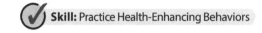 **Skill:** Practice Health-Enhancing Behaviors

Classroom Energizer

Instructions: *A classroom energizer is a short physical activity routine that all students can do together in a classroom. Create a five-minute classroom energizer that incorporates at least five components of health-related and skill-related fitness. Share your routine with the class.*

1. Physical activity: _____

   A. Time: _____

   B. Health-related fitness component(s) demonstrated: _____

   _____

   C. Skill-related fitness component(s) demonstrated: _____

   _____

2. Physical activity: _____

   A. Time: _____

   B. Health-related fitness component(s) demonstrated: _____

   _____

   C. Skill-related fitness component(s) demonstrated: _____

   _____

3. Physical activity: _____

   A. Time: _____

   B. Health-related fitness component(s) demonstrated: _____

   _____

   C. Skill-related fitness component(s) demonstrated: _____

   _____

4. Physical activity: _____

   A. Time: _____

   B. Health-related fitness component(s) demonstrated: _____

   _____

   C. Skill-related fitness component(s) demonstrated: _____

   _____

5. Physical activity: _____

   A. Time: _____

   B. Health-related fitness component(s) demonstrated: _____
   _____

   C. Skill-related fitness component(s) demonstrated: _____
   _____

6. Physical activity: _____

   A. Time: _____

   B. Health-related fitness component(s) demonstrated: _____
   _____

   C. Skill-related fitness component(s) demonstrated: _____
   _____

7. Physical activity: _____

   A. Time: _____

   B. Health-related fitness component(s) demonstrated: _____
   _____

   C. Skill-related fitness component(s) demonstrated: _____
   _____

8. Physical activity: _____

   A. Time: _____

   B. Health-related fitness component(s) demonstrated: _____
   _____

   C. Skill-related fitness component(s) demonstrated: _____
   _____

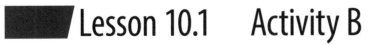 Lesson 10.1   Activity B

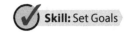

Building Fitness

Instructions: *Read the following scenarios and write a long-term SMART goal that uses health-related or skill-related fitness to help each person achieve better physical health. Then, write two short-term goals that will help break up this long-term goal into more manageable parts.*

Scenario 1

> Leilani loves to dance, and used to do ballet when she was little. While she does not want to compete in dance anymore, she likes to do dance-based fitness classes like Zumba or barre to maintain her flexibility and balance.

1. Long-term SMART goal: _____

_____

2. Short-term goals: _____

_____

_____

_____

Scenario 2

> Charlie has played baseball every summer since he was seven, but playing in high school is on a new level for him. Playing at third base, Charlie is struggling to learn how to field bunts and other in-field hits properly. His teammates seem to be more agile and coordinated than he is.

1. Long-term SMART goal: _____

_____

2. Short-term goals: _____

_____

_____

_____

Scenario 3

> Demi loves when she works hard at her strength training and sees her muscle strength increase. Demi has also seen a vast improvement in the power of her strikes in volleyball and thinks she might make the varsity team next year if she keeps working at it.

1. Long-term SMART goal: _____

_____

2. Short-term goals: _____

_____

_____

_____

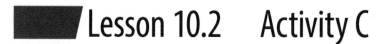 Lesson 10.2   Activity C   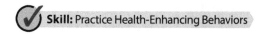 **Skill:** Practice Health-Enhancing Behaviors

Charting Your Physical Activity

Instructions: *Track your physical activity for one week to assess how well you currently meet the recommended amount of physical activity (one hour per day). Then, answer the questions that follow.*

Tracking Physical Activity

1. How much time did you spend on physical activity?

   A. Day 1: _____   E. Day 5: _____

   B. Day 2: _____   F. Day 6: _____

   C. Day 3: _____   G. Day 7: _____

   D. Day 4: _____

2. How much time did you spend on sedentary activities?

   A. Day 1: _____   E. Day 5: _____

   B. Day 2: _____   F. Day 6: _____

   C. Day 3: _____   G. Day 7: _____

   D. Day 4: _____

3. Calculate the total time active. _____

4. Calculate the total time sedentary. _____

Questions

5. Were you successful in engaging in one hour of physical activity each day? Explain your answer.

   _____

   _____

6. What obstacles (if any) did you experience in achieving an hour of physical activity? What did you do to overcome these obstacles?

   _____

   _____

7. On the days you engaged in physical activity, reflect on how you felt during and after the activity. Describe any physical, mental and emotional, and social benefits.

   _____

   _____

8. What can you do to increase the amount of physical activity you get each day? Be specific.

   _____

   _____

9. Reflect on the sedentary activities you engaged in each day. Can you reduce any sedentary activities in your daily schedule? Explain your answer.

   _____

   _____

Lesson 10.2   Activity D

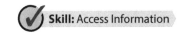
Skill: Access Information

Fitness That Fits You

Instructions: *Research the different fitness methods listed. For each method of fitness, fill in the required information. Once you have filled in the information and researched each method thoroughly, answer the question that follows.*

Fitness Methods

1. Weight lifting

   A. Equipment required: _____

   B. Cost: _____

   C. Time needed: _____

   D. Group-oriented or solitary: _____

2. Jogging, walking, or running

   A. Equipment required: _____

   B. Cost: _____

   C. Time needed: _____

   D. Group-oriented or solitary: _____

3. Organized sport

   A. Equipment required: _____

   B. Cost: _____

   C. Time needed: _____

   D. Group-oriented or solitary: _____

4. At-home fitness video

   A. Equipment required: _____

   B. Cost: _____

   C. Time needed: _____

   D. Group-oriented or solitary: _____

5. Other: _____

   A. Equipment required: _____

   B. Cost: _____

   C. Time needed: _____

   D. Group-oriented or solitary: _____

Question

6. Do any of these fitness activities "fit" for you? Explain why or why not.

   _____

   _____

   _____

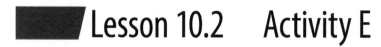 Lesson 10.2   Activity E

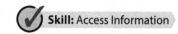

Being Active in Your Community

Instructions: *Many schools and communities provide free or low-cost ways to enjoy physical activities. Research four convenient places to get physical activity in your community that meet your desired fitness needs. Organize your information below. Then, answer the reflection questions.*

Places to Get Physical Activity

1. Place in the community to get physical activity: _____

    A. Cost: _____

    B. Type of physical activity: _____

2. Place in the community to get physical activity: _____

    A. Cost: _____

    B. Type of physical activity: _____

3. Place in the community to get physical activity: _____

    A. Cost: _____

    B. Type of physical activity: _____

4. Place in the community to get physical activity: _____

    A. Cost: _____

    B. Type of physical activity: _____

Questions

5. Do you like to be physically active alone or with other people? Based on this answer, which place or places in your community would be ideal for you to get physical activity?

    _____

    _____

    _____

    _____

6. Based on your family situation, transportation, money available, and convenience, which place would be realistic for you to be physically active on a regular basis? Defend your answer.

    _____

    _____

    _____

    _____

7. Describe your ideal place to get physical activity. What makes it ideal?

    _____

    _____

    _____

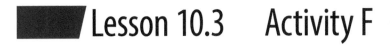 Lesson 10.3   Activity F   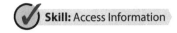 **Skill:** Access Information

Be a Smart Fitness Consumer

Instructions: *Many physical activities require fitness equipment or products. For each product or equipment listed below, research studies about a popular brand. Assess whether each piece of equipment or product is as effective or as safe as its company might claim. Use reliable resources and provide the citations for each source.*

1. Football helmets

   A. The brand: _____

   B. Claims made about this product: _____
   _____
   _____

   C. Scientific research about effectiveness or safety: _____
   _____
   _____
   _____

   D. Citation for reliable resource: _____

2. Running shoes

   A. The brand: _____

   B. Claims made about this product: _____
   _____
   _____

   C. Scientific research about effectiveness or safety: _____
   _____
   _____
   _____

   D. Citation for reliable resource: _____

3. Sports drinks

   A. The brand: _____

   B. Claims made about this product: _____
   _____
   _____

   C. Scientific research about effectiveness or safety: _____
   _____
   _____
   _____

   D. Citation for reliable resource: _____

Lesson 10.3   Activity G

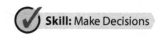

Rewrite the Story

Instructions: *Read the following scenarios and identify mistakes that jeopardize each person's safety. Then, rewrite the stories by changing the mistakes and adding safety tips.*

Scenario 1

On Saturday morning, Oliver gets a text from his friends that they are playing soccer at the neighborhood park. Oliver quickly runs out the door, jumps on his bike, and pedals to the park. While playing, one of his friends bumps into him and Oliver hits his head on the ground. He sits out for a few minutes, but then gets back to playing. He feels a little dizzy riding his bike home.

1. What two mistakes did Oliver make that jeopardized his personal safety?

_____

_____

2. Rewrite Oliver's story so that he does not make these mistakes and he returns home safely.

_____

_____

_____

_____

_____

_____

Scenario 2

On a hot summer afternoon, Malika decides to run six miles. She recently started working out and has never run more than two miles in a row. Malika dresses in two pairs of dark sweatpants and a dark sweatshirt to increase sweat on her run and does not bring water with her. After fifty minutes of running, Malika begins to feel sick.

1. What three mistakes did Malika make that jeopardized her personal safety?

_____

_____

2. Rewrite Malika's story so that she does not make these mistakes and she returns home safely.

_____

_____

_____

_____

_____

_____

Name _____ Date _____ Period _____

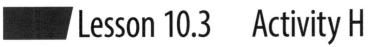 Lesson 10.3   Activity H

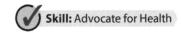

In the News

Instructions: *Read the following scenario about an opportunity to advocate for the health of your community.*

A high-poverty neighborhood in your community is in need of warm clothes and outerwear during the winter months when temperatures are as low as 17 degrees. This community encourages outdoor exercise year-round to increase positive interactions and decrease crime rates. Your community is looking to collect clothing donations or raise money to purchase warm clothes and outerwear for the kids.

Instructions: *Write an article for your school newspaper suggesting a cold-weather clothing campaign. Answer the following questions in your article.*

1. Which two cold-related health conditions are the kids in this neighborhood at risk of developing? What are the symptoms of these conditions?

_____

_____

_____

_____

_____

_____

2. What type of clothing can protect the kids from these conditions?

_____

_____

_____

_____

_____

3. What strategies can people implement to stay safe during cold temperatures? (Name four.)

A. Strategy: _____

_____

_____

B. Strategy: _____

_____

_____

C. Strategy: _____

_____

_____

D. Strategy: _____

_____

4. What kind of campaign can your community implement to help? What ideas do you have?

_____

_____

_____

_____

_____

_____

5. Write your article here.

_____

_____

_____

_____

_____

_____

_____

_____

_____

_____

_____

_____

_____

_____

_____

_____

_____

_____

_____

_____

_____

_____

_____

_____

_____

_____

_____

_____

_____

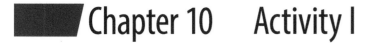 Chapter 10   Activity I

Practice Test

Completion

Instructions: *Write the term that completes the statement in the space provided.*

1. _____ activities use oxygen to break down energy for use in the muscles.

   _____

2. Many people spend much of their day engaging in _____ behaviors rather than physical activity.

   _____

3. The acronym FITT stands for frequency, _____, time, and type.

   _____

4. The _____ principle states that you must put demands on your body to improve it.

   _____

5. Loss of fluid through sweat can lead to _____ if a person does not drink enough water before, during, and after physical activity.

   _____

True/False

Instructions: *Indicate whether each statement below is true or false.*

6. _____ *True or false?* People who engage in regular physical activity experience a better quality of sleep than those who do not exercise.

7. _____ *True or false?* Muscular strength is the ability of a muscle to exert force against resistance.

8. _____ *True or false?* Skill-related fitness means fitness that is used to perform daily activities with ease and energy.

9. _____ *True or false?* The *Physical Activity Guidelines for Americans* suggests teens get at least two hours of physical activity every day.

10. _____ *True or false?* Warming up before physical activity can help prevent injuries.

Multiple Choice

Instructions: *Select the letter that corresponds to the correct answer.*

11. _____ The body's ability to perform daily activities and meet unexpected physical demands is _____.
    A. flexibility   C. agility
    B. physical fitness   D. exercise

12. _____ Which of the following is a combination of strength and speed?
    A. coordination   C. balance
    B. agility   D. power

13. _____ An effective fitness program should _____.
    A. consist of the same types of physical activity   C. match up well with your daily life and interests
    B. be far too difficult for your current level of   D. be kept private from your friends or family
       fitness

14. _____ An easy way to monitor the intensity of physical activity is to check your _____.
    A. pulse   C. breathing
    B. sweat levels   D. endurance

15. _____ Although water and sports drinks help you stay hydrated, _____ also provides carbohydrates and proteins to help build and repair muscles.
   A. soda
   B. chocolate milk
   C. an energy drink
   D. coffee

Matching

Instructions: *Match each key term to its definition (16–22).*

16. _____ number of heartbeats per minute that is safe and effective for a given intensity

17. _____ three health conditions related to intense physical activity in females

18. _____ activities that consist of sitting or lying down and using very little energy

19. _____ abnormal absence of menstrual period

20. _____ number of heartbeats per minute when the heart is working its hardest

21. _____ recommendations about how much physical activity children, teens, and adults should get

22. _____ brain chemicals that improve mood; released during physical activity

A. amenorrhea
B. endorphins
C. female athlete triad
D. maximum heart rate
E. Physical Activity Guidelines for Americans
F. sedentary behaviors
G. target heart rate

Analyzing Data

Instructions: *The following chart presents World Health Organization statistics on physical inactivity around the world. Study the data in this chart and answer the questions that follow.*

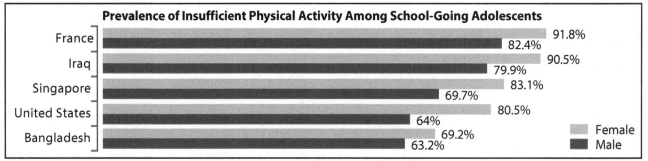

Figure 1. Percentage of physical inactivity among school-going adolescents around the world

23. What percentage of teen females in the US get enough physical activity? How does this rate compare to teen males in the US?

_____

24. If there are two million teen males in France, how many are currently getting enough physical activity?

_____

25. How do the rates of physical inactivity for females in Bangladesh compare to those in Iraq? for males?

_____

Short Answer

Instructions: *Answer the following question using what you have learned in this chapter.*

26. What are some simple ways that you can incorporate more physical activity into your daily life? Remember that physical activity does not have to be structured.

_____

_____

_____

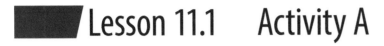

CHAPTER 11 / Vaping and Tobacco

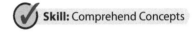

Lesson 11.1   Activity A   ✓ **Skill:** Comprehend Concepts

Tobacco and Your Body Systems

Instructions: *Answer the following questions based on the information in this lesson. If needed, you may also refer to Background Lesson 1, "The Body Systems," in your textbook.*

The Impact of Nicotine

1. Nicotine triggers the release of adrenaline. What negative impact does this have on the cardiovascular system?

_____

_____

_____

_____

_____

_____

2. What chemical, released by the brain in response to nicotine, leads to a pleasurable sensation? Explain how this sensation is associated with addiction.

_____

_____

_____

_____

_____

_____

_____

_____

_____

_____

Health Effects of Cigarettes

1. List four chemicals found in cigarette smoke and describe what other substances typically contain these chemicals.

_____

_____

_____

2. What three respiratory diseases combine in chronic obstructive pulmonary disease? How does smoking cause this disease?

_____

_____

_____

_____

_____

_____

Health Effects of Vaping

1. Why might you not know what chemicals are in your vaping e-liquid?

_____

_____

_____

_____

2. How can ingredients in e-liquids be dangerous to inhale, even if the Food and Drug Administration deems them *generally recognized as safe*?

_____

_____

_____

_____

3. Which rare lung disease is related to the presence of diacetyl in e-liquid? How does diacetyl cause this disease?

_____

_____

_____

_____

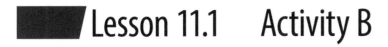 # Lesson 11.1   Activity B

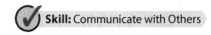 Skill: Communicate with Others

Identifying the Stages of Substance Use

Instructions: *Identify which stage of substance use is described in each of the following scenarios. In the space provided, write a short note to each person. Describe health conditions for which they are at risk. Communicate the information in a way that shows respect to the other person.*

Scenario 1

Celeste used to vape a few times a week, and for a long time that seemed like enough. Now, however, Celeste notices that a hit of her vape does not satisfy her for as long as it used to. She is starting to vape before classes, during lunch, after her last class, and when doing her homework in the evenings.

1. Stage of substance use: _____

2. Write a note to Celeste. _____

_____

Scenario 2

Javier is a catcher on his baseball team, and at baseball games, Javier sometimes sees some players chewing tobacco and spitting in the dugout. He is curious and asks if he can try some.

1. Stage of substance use: _____

2. Write a note to Javier. _____

_____

Scenario 3

Justin smokes when he feels stressed-out, usually following an argument with his parents or after a particularly difficult day at school. He feels that smoking relaxes him. Lately, however, he has noticed that he needs to smoke two cigarettes to get the same relaxed feeling he used to get after only smoking one.

1. Stage of substance use: _____

2. Write a note to Justin. _____

_____

Scenario 4

After smoking regularly for a year, Hannah decides to quit. Going without cigarettes is harder than she thought. After only a few days, she feels jittery, irritable, and sick to her stomach. She frequently experiences intense cravings for cigarettes. Hannah fears she will never feel like her "normal" self without them.

1. Stage of substance use: _____

2. Write a note to Hannah. _____

_____

Lesson 11.1   Activity C

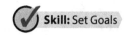

Making a Tobacco-Free Pledge

Instructions: *Developing a goal to remain tobacco-free can help you maintain or improve your personal health practices. Design a tobacco-free pledge that you would sign by responding to the following statements. Do additional research as needed.*

1. List two harmful effects of nicotine on your personal health.

   _____

   _____

2. List two harmful effects of vaping on your personal health.

   _____

   _____

3. List two harmful effects of smokeless tobacco on your personal health.

   _____

   _____

4. Identify one mental consequence of tobacco use.

   _____

5. Identify one social consequence of tobacco use.

   _____

6. Identify one legal consequence of tobacco use.

   _____

7. List two harmful effects of secondhand smoke and aerosol on others.

   _____

   _____

8. Provide an inspirational quote.

   _____

   _____

9. Name an example of a role model who is tobacco-free.

   _____

10. Create a SMART goal that will help you remain tobacco-free. (Remember to make this goal specific, measurable, achievable, relevant, and timely.)

    _____

    _____

11. State your pledge.

    _____

    _____

    _____

Name _____ Date _____ Period _____

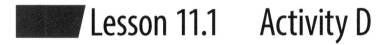 Lesson 11.1   Activity D

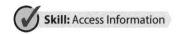

Myths About Tobacco Use

Instructions: *Read the following statements about tobacco use. Research the truth behind these statements. Be sure to use credible, up-to-date resources. Record the scientific research around each statement, and cite your reliable source. Then, answer the question below.*

Statements

1. Using tobacco only occasionally is not dangerous.
   A. Record your scientific findings.

   _____

   _____

   _____

   B. Cite the resource used.

   _____

2. Vaping devices emit water vapor rather than smoke.
   A. Record your scientific findings.

   _____

   _____

   _____

   B. Cite the resource used.

   _____

3. There is no point in someone who uses tobacco quitting since the damage has already been done.
   A. Record your scientific findings.

   _____

   _____

   _____

   B. Cite the resource used.

   _____

4. Secondhand smoke and aerosol are more bothersome than dangerous.
   A. Record your scientific findings.

   _____

   _____

   _____

   B. Cite the resource used.

   _____

5. Smoking by an open window can prevent secondhand smoke.
   A. Record your scientific findings.

   _____

   _____

   _____

   B. Cite the resource used.

   _____

6. Light or low-tar cigarettes are less dangerous than regular cigarettes.
   A. Record your scientific findings.

   _____

   _____

   _____

   B. Cite the resource used.

   _____

7. Using nicotine replacement is just as dangerous as using tobacco.
   A. Record your scientific findings.

   _____

   _____

   _____

   B. Cite the resource used.

   _____

8. Quitting tobacco can worsen mental health conditions.
   A. Record your scientific findings.

   _____

   _____

   _____

   B. Cite the resource used.

   _____

9. Medical advances have decreased the risk of developing tobacco-related cancers in recent decades.
   A. Record your scientific findings.

   _____

   _____

   _____

   B. Cite the resource used.

   _____

Question

1. How do you think common statements such as those provided here affect how people think about tobacco use?

   _____

   _____

Name _____ Date _____ Period _____

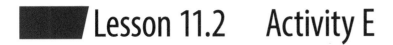 Lesson 11.2 Activity E

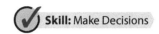

Can This Friendship Be Saved?

Instructions: *Asia and Lena have been best friends since third grade. Now they are both in the tenth grade and go to the same high school. Lena recently began vaping, which has led to tension in their relationship. For each of the following situations, describe what you think Asia should do. Then explain why you think Asia and Lena's friendship can or cannot be saved.*

Situation 1

In the morning, Asia picks up Lena at her house and gives her a ride to school. Lena uses her vape pen in the car. Asia does not like the way the vape makes her cough. She knows that breathing secondhand aerosol can affect her health.

1. What should Asia say or do?_____

_____

Situation 2

Lena and Asia used to have lunch together in the cafeteria, but now Lena wants to go off campus during lunch breaks so she can vape. Lena hitches a ride with her new vaping friends and wants Asia to come along.

1. What should Asia say or do?_____

_____

Situation 3

Lena's parents do not know that she vapes. Lena says that if they knew, she would be grounded for life. One day, Asia goes to Lena's house after school, and Lena vapes continuously while they play a game. When Lena's father comes home, he asks about the vape pen on the table. Lena says, "Oh, that's just a USB drive that Asia uses for her homework—right, Asia?" Asia respects Lena's father and could get grounded by her own parents for lying.

1. What should Asia say or do?_____

_____

Situation 4

Now that she vapes, Lena is spending more and more time hanging out with other teenagers who vape. Lena invites Asia to a party where she can meet her new friends. When Asia arrives, everyone is vaping, including Lena. "Come on, Asia, have a puff," says Lena as she tries to hand Asia a vape pen. Lena's new friends chime in, "Yeah, it won't bite you!" Asia feels all their eyes on her and she wants desperately to fit in.

1. What should Asia say or do?_____

_____

Question

1. Based on the situations above, summarize how Lena's vaping is impacting Asia and their friendship. Do you think the girls can or should remain best friends? Why or why not?

_____

_____

Lesson 11.2   Activity F

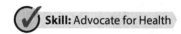 Skill: Advocate for Health

You Be the Government

Instructions: *Read the following scenario in small groups. For each question below, describe what you and your group can do realistically to solve the issue.*

> Imagine that you have been elected to a public health advisory board in a small country. Together, you plan to improve education, clean up polluted waterways, and improve food production and safety. Your programs will cost millions of dollars that your country does not have because so much money is being spent on healthcare. Healthcare costs are high in part because so many people use tobacco products, including cigarettes and vaping devices. Each year, several million people receive healthcare for serious diseases caused by tobacco use or receive treatment for nicotine addictions. Even though your government has limited control over private businesses, your advisory board decides your government must do all it can to eliminate tobacco use.

1. What laws and regulations can your government implement to limit the marketing and advertising of tobacco products?

_____

_____

2. What laws and regulations can your government implement to limit the sale of tobacco products?

_____

_____

3. What can your government do to limit the public's exposure to secondhand smoke and aerosol?

_____

_____

_____

_____

4. What can your government do to educate the public about the dangers of tobacco use?

_____

_____

_____

_____

5. What can your government do to help people with a nicotine addiction quit using tobacco products?

_____

_____

_____

_____

6. What laws and regulations can your government implement to regulate the price of tobacco products?

_____

_____

_____

_____

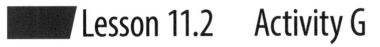 **Lesson 11.2   Activity G**   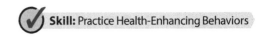 **Skill:** Practice Health-Enhancing Behaviors

Resisting Peer Pressure

Instructions: *Read the following scenarios about your peers who feel pressured to use tobacco products. With a partner, discuss factors that are influencing Noah, Harper, Ana, and Reza to want to use tobacco products. Talk about what they can do to resist this pressure. Choose one scenario and act it out for the class, demonstrating the strategies used to maintain personal health.*

Scenario 1

Noah and his best friend Logan are hanging out after school, waiting for their bus to arrive. While waiting outside, a classmate offers them a hit on his vape pen. Logan surprises Noah by accepting the vape. Noah says "no thanks," but Logan and the classmate roll their eyes at each other and continue to vape without him. Noah does not want them to tease him, and he does not think it would be too harmful to do it just this once.

1. What behaviors can help Noah resist the pressure to vape?

_____

_____

Scenario 2

Harper is very close with her older cousin, Amber, and has always been welcome to hang out with her friends. These older girls are cool, and Harper loves spending time with them. Lately, they have started smoking a hookah in Amber's basement. Harper does not want to try it, but every time she says "no," she worries they will stop wanting her to hang out with them.

1. What behaviors can help Harper resist the pressure to smoke?

_____

_____

Scenario 3

It is tradition at Ana's high school for seniors to smoke cigarillos in the parking lot after class. Initially, Ana thought it sounded like a dumb and gross tradition. Every day, however, she watches her friends laugh and smoke together. The cigarillos smell fruity, too, and not disgusting like regular cigarettes.

1. What behaviors can help Ana resist the pressure to smoke?

_____

_____

Scenario 4

It seems like everyone in Reza's family smokes one form of tobacco or another. His dad smokes cigars, his mom prefers cigarettes, and his grandpa puffs on a pipe at night. Reza's sister told him that smoking like that can cause cancer and asthma and explained that is why she vapes instead. She told him she would teach him how to use her vape pen if he wanted.

1. What behaviors can help Reza resist the pressure to vape?

_____

_____

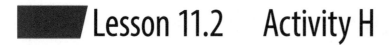 Lesson 11.2   Activity H

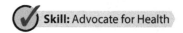

Create an Anti-Vaping Advertisement

Instructions: *In small groups, create an anti-vaping advertisement to convince people to stop vaping or never begin vaping. Follow the instructions below to get started. Then create your advertisement, using the medium of your choice, and share it with the class.*

Choose a target group.

1. Advertisements are crafted to appeal to a particular audience. Which group(s) of people will your anti-vaping advertisement target? Some target audiences might be teenagers, adults, women or men, people of a particular economic or ethnic group, or people who do or do not vape. Describe your target audience.

_____

_____

_____

_____

_____

_____

Choose a focus.

1. Choose an anti-vaping message you want to communicate. "Vaping is bad" is too broad. You should choose a narrower focus. For example, you might focus on the addictive nature of e-liquids or the fact that vaping can cause respiratory conditions. Consider what kind of anti-vaping message will appeal to the group you have chosen. Summarize the message of your ad in one or two sentences.

_____

_____

_____

_____

_____

_____

Choose a medium for your message.

1. Choose a medium for your advertisement. Your group might create a flyer, a poster, a video, a podcast, or a website. When choosing your medium, consider which medium will best reach your target audience. Describe which medium your group chose and why you chose it.

_____

_____

_____

_____

_____

_____

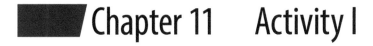 **Chapter 11   Activity I**

Practice Test

Completion

Instructions: *Write the term that completes the statement in the space provided.*

1. _____ devices heat tobacco or synthetic nicotine without burning it.

   _____

2. People who use nicotine show more _____ in their skin.

   _____

3. Carbon monoxide in cigarette smoke interferes with the ability of blood cells to carry _____.

   _____

4. Vaping introduces the addictive, dangerous substance _____ into a person's body.

   _____

5. Living or socializing with people who smoke or vape increases rates of cancer because of _____ smoke or aerosol.

   _____

True/False

Instructions: *Indicate whether each statement below is true or false.*

6. _____ *True or false?* Smoking is the leading cause of preventable death in the United States.

7. _____ *True or false?* Tobacco smoke contains more than 70 carcinogens.

8. _____ *True or false?* Most people who smoke picked up the habit as adults.

9. _____ *True or false?* Most people who have had a heart attack or surgery resulting from lung cancer stop smoking.

10. _____ *True or false?* Stimulus control helps people respond to difficult feelings and situations with stress management, relaxation, and coping skills instead of tobacco use.

Multiple Choice

Instructions: *Select the letter that corresponds to the correct answer.*

11. _____ Nicotine triggers the release of adrenaline, which causes a(n) _____.
    A. pleasurable sensation   C. increase in blood pressure
    B. reduction in fertility   D. greater risk of illness

12. _____ Which chemical leads to a pleasurable sensation when released in the brain, such as in response to nicotine?
    A. adrenaline   C. benzene
    B. insulin   D. dopamine

13. _____ People who smoke are at greater risk of becoming ill from germs that cause colds and the flu due to a weakened _____.
    A. respiratory system   C. heart
    B. immune system   D. lung capacity

14. _____ A laryngectomy is performed on people, often people who have smoked, who have _____.
    A. lung cancer   C. heart disease
    B. cancer of the larynx   D. oral cancer

15. _____ How long after quitting smoking will people see their heart rate, blood pressure, and circulation return to normal?
- A. one hour
- B. one week
- C. one year
- D. 10 years

Matching

Instructions: *Match each key term to its definition (16–23).*

16. _____ particles and gases left over after someone smokes a cigarette; remains on surfaces nearby

17. _____ condition that damages the lungs' smallest airways; leads to coughing and shortness of breath

18. _____ condition characterized by thickened, white, leathery spots inside the mouth; can develop into oral cancer

19. _____ tobacco product that is chewed or snuffed rather than smoked

20. _____ tobacco products that heat tobacco or synthetic nicotine without burning it, producing an aerosol

21. _____ treatment for nicotine addiction that involves avoiding tempting situations and managing feelings that lead to nicotine use

22. _____ treatment for nicotine addiction where people practice responding to difficult feelings and situations using stress management, relaxation, and coping skills instead of tobacco use

23. _____ treatment for nicotine addiction that continues to put some nicotine into the body; lessens withdrawal symptoms and cravings, making it easier to quit

- A. leukoplakia
- B. nicotine replacement
- C. popcorn lung
- D. response substitution
- E. smokeless tobacco
- F. stimulus control
- G. thirdhand smoke
- H. vaping devices

Analyzing Data

Instructions: *Read the data from the Centers for Disease Control and Prevention below to answer the following questions.*

Vaping Among Students 2017–2019

Middle school students: 3.3 (2017), 4.9 (2018), 10.5 (2019)

High school students: 11.7 (2017), 20.8 (2018), 27.7 (2019)

Legend: 2017, 2018, 2019

Centers for Disease Control and Prevention

Figure 1. Percentage of vaping among middle school and high school students

24. For which group of students was vaping more popular? _____

25. How much did vaping rates increase between 2017 and 2019 for high school students? _____

Short Answer

Instructions: *Answer the following questions using what you have learned in this chapter.*

26. How does peer pressure influence decisions about tobacco use positively? negatively?

_____

_____

27. Some researchers believe that the best way to prevent teenagers from using tobacco is to emphasize the negative effects of tobacco use on appearance and hygiene. Do you agree or disagree? Explain your answer.

_____

_____

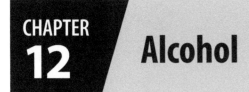

CHAPTER 12 / **Alcohol**

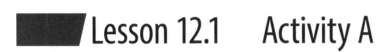 Lesson 12.1 Activity A

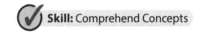 **Skill:** Comprehend Concepts

Alcohol and the Brain

Instructions: *Identify the functions of each part of the brain. Also, describe the impairments caused by alcohol that affect each of those parts. Then, answer the questions that follow about long-term brain damage from alcohol.*

Immediate Effects

1. Cerebral cortex

   A. What does this part of the brain do? _____

   B. What are the immediate effects of alcohol on this part of the brain?

   _____

2. Cerebellum

   A. What does this part of the brain do? _____

   B. What are the immediate effects of alcohol on this part of the brain?

   _____

3. Hippocampus

   A. What does this part of the brain do? _____

   B. What are the immediate effects of alcohol on this part of the brain?

   _____

4. Hypothalamus and pituitary gland

   A. What do these parts of the brain do? _____

   B. What are the immediate effects of alcohol on these parts of the brain?

   _____

5. Medulla

   A. What does this part of the brain do? _____

   B. What are the immediate effects of alcohol on this part of the brain?

   _____

Long-Term Damage

1. List three neurological conditions people might experience if they drink heavily or binge-drink on a regular basis.

   _____

2. How can alcohol use among teens permanently affect the white matter of the brain and the prefrontal cortex?

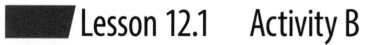 ## Lesson 12.1   Activity B

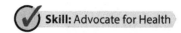

The Effects of Underage Drinking

Instructions: *Read the following scenarios and determine the consequences of drinking alcohol for each teen.*

1. Samantha's sister is annoyed with her because her drinking has gotten in the way of their old movie night tradition. Samantha has been missing more and more movie nights since she started hanging out with a new group of friends and began drinking.

   A. Explain the impact on Samantha's physical health, education, social life, or future.

   _____

   _____

   _____

2. Ben was charged with a DUI and had his license suspended. Not being able to drive in the evenings means that he cannot get to his part-time job at a local fast-food restaurant. He has been saving up money for college, but now he may lose his job.

   A. Explain the impact on Ben's physical health, education, social life, or future.

   _____

   _____

   _____

3. Devon started hanging out with a new group of friends, and now he often spends his evenings drinking with them. As a result, he has missed several football practices. The coach cannot afford to have a player who does not pull his weight. He cuts Devon from the team.

   A. Explain the impact on Devon's physical health, education, social life, or future.

   _____

   _____

   _____

4. Kiki's habit of having a few drinks on the weekends with her friends has gotten out of hand. Now she has been drinking on school nights, and the hangovers she has in the mornings make it hard to concentrate in class. Recently, she failed an important test in her math class.

   A. Explain the impact on Kiki's physical health, education, social life, or future.

   _____

   _____

   _____

5. Julian spent a Saturday drinking with his friends and he knew he was too intoxicated to drive home. Instead, he walked home, but the weather was very cold that evening. As a result, Julian caught a bad cold and had to stay home from school for several days.

   A. Explain the impact on Julian's physical health, education, social life, or future.

   _____

   _____

   _____

Instructions: *In small groups, using the negative impacts identified in the scenarios above, create a campaign to present the consequences of underage drinking to students at your school. This campaign can use whatever medium you choose, such as social media posts, posters, emails, presentations, or flyers.*

Name _____ Date _____ Period _____

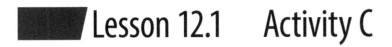 Lesson 12.1   Activity C   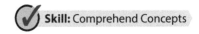 **Skill:** Comprehend Concepts

Level of Intoxication

Instructions: *Study the information in this activity about how much alcohol is in each type of drink. Then, use this information to answer the questions. For each scenario presented, determine how many ounces of alcohol each person has drunk, how much of that alcohol each person has processed, and who is the most intoxicated by the time everyone goes home.*

Processing Alcohol

The liver can process between .25 and .50 ounces of alcohol each hour. In the scenarios that follow, assume that everyone is processing alcohol at .30 ounces per hour.

Alcohol Content Guide

0.6 ounces of pure alcohol is equal to:

- 12 ounces of beer, hard cider, hard lemonade, or hard seltzer
- 5 ounces of wine
- 8 ounces malt liquor
- 1.5 ounces of liquor, such as rum, vodka, tequila, or whiskey

Scenarios

1. Kate, Luka, and Stacy have been drinking together for three hours. Over the past three hours, Kate has drunk two glasses of beer. Luka has drunk three shots of vodka and a glass of beer. Stacy has drunk one and a half glasses of malt liquor.

    A. How many ounces of alcohol have Kate, Luka, and Stacy drunk?

    Kate: _____

    Luka: _____

    Stacy: _____

    B. How many ounces of alcohol do they process in three hours?

    Kate: _____

    Luka: _____

    Stacy: _____

    C. How many ounces of alcohol are left unprocessed?

    Kate: _____

    Luka: _____

    Stacy: _____

    D. Who is the most intoxicated? _____

2. Bakari and Jane arrived at the bar two hours ago. Bakari has drunk two shots of vodka and a glass of malt liquor. Jane has drunk one beer.

    A. How many ounces of alcohol have Bakari and Jane drunk?

    Bakari: _____

    Jane: _____

B. How many ounces of alcohol do they process in two hours?

Bakari: _____

Jane: _____

C. How many ounces of alcohol are left unprocessed?

Bakari: _____

Jane: _____

D. Who is the most intoxicated? _____

3. Wine is being served at this week's book discussion hour. In that hour, Lauren has drunk three glasses of wine, Andrea has drunk one glass, and Jerome has drunk half of one glass.

A. How many ounces of alcohol have Lauren, Andrea, and Jerome drunk?

Lauren: _____

Andrea: _____

Jerome: _____

B. How many ounces of alcohol do they process in one hour?

Lauren: _____

Andrea: _____

Jerome: _____

C. How many ounces of alcohol are left unprocessed?

Lauren: _____

Andrea: _____

Jerome: _____

D. Who is the most intoxicated? _____

4. Marco is at a bachelor party for his friend Derek. During the past six hours of partying, Marco has drunk three beers and two shots of vodka. Derek has drunk six beers and four shots of vodka.

A. How many ounces of alcohol have Marco and Derek drunk?

Marco: _____

Derek: _____

B. How many ounces of alcohol do they process six hours?

Marco: _____

Derek: _____

C. How many ounces of alcohol are left unprocessed?

Marco: _____

Derek: _____

D. Who is the most intoxicated? _____

Question

5. In the previous scenarios, it is assumed that the factors affecting the blood alcohol concentration (BAC) were equal for each person. Besides how much a person drinks in a certain amount of time, list four factors that can influence BAC.

_____

_____

_____

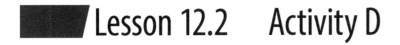 Lesson 12.2   Activity D   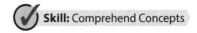 **Skill:** Comprehend Concepts

The Voice of Reason

Instructions: *Intoxication from alcohol can impair judgment in ways that result in violence or serious injury. For each scenario, serve as the "voice of reason" and write how you would stop the situations from getting out of hand and keep your friends safe.*

1. You are hanging out at your friend Grayson's house on a Friday evening. Grayson has been drinking, but you have not. All night, Grayson has been expressing worry about his poor grades and his fear that he will not be able to graduate. As he continues to drink, Grayson gets more and more depressed and even mentions thoughts of suicide.

   A. What would you say?

   _____

   _____

   _____

   _____

2. You and your friend Jenny have been watching movies and it is now very late. Jenny has been drinking, but you have not. Jenny's family has a pool in their backyard and she announces that she would like to go swimming. Jenny sneaks outside to the pool and you follow her. You know that swimming can be a dangerous activity if she is intoxicated and not in full control of her actions.

   A. What would you say?

   _____

   _____

   _____

   _____

3. You and a few friends are hanging out in Jared's backyard and have started a bonfire. Although most of the people there are drinking, you and a few friends are not. Everyone seems to be having fun at first, but then you hear someone shout angrily. Before you know it, two of your friends who were drinking are shouting at each other and squaring off as though they are going to fight.

   A. What would you say?

   _____

   _____

   _____

   _____

4. You are hanging out with friends who are drinking casually, but you have chosen not to drink. You notice that your friend Beth is drinking more than anyone else. By the end of the evening, Beth has passed out on the couch and has already vomited once. You are worried that Beth may have alcohol poisoning, but no one else seems concerned.

   A. What would you say?

   _____

   _____

   _____

   _____

Lesson 12.2   Activity E

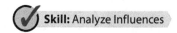

Nature or Nurture

Instructions: *In the following scenarios, determine which factor—nature (genes) or nurture (environment)— influences a person's alcohol use, and identify two ways the person can avoid the temptation to drink alcohol. Keep in mind that often, nature and nurture both influence alcohol use.*

1. Becky has grown up surrounded by alcohol at family gatherings during the holidays. When she begins celebrating the holidays—or any occasion—on her own, she also includes alcohol in the festivities.

   A. Nature or Nurture? _____

   B. List strategies for avoiding alcohol.

   _____

   _____

2. Growing up, Terrance's biological father would yell and become irrationally angry. Years later, Terrance's older brother explained that their father had an alcohol use disorder. When Terrance drinks, he often yells and becomes angry as well.

   A. Nature or Nurture? _____

   B. List strategies for avoiding alcohol.

   _____

   _____

3. Violet was never interested in drinking growing up and there was not much alcohol in her home. When she started high school, however, Violet began hanging out with new friends who drank more often. Soon, Violet began drinking regularly with her friends.

   A. Nature or Nurture? _____

   B. List strategies for avoiding alcohol.

   _____

   _____

4. Rosie and Caryn are twins. When the girls were in high school, Rosie often spent her weekends drinking with friends, sometimes to the point of abusing alcohol. Later, when the twins went to college, Caryn began drinking and abusing alcohol as well.

   A. Nature or Nurture? _____

   B. List strategies for avoiding alcohol.

   _____

   _____

5. Neither of Lincoln's parents drink, nor do his older siblings. However, Lincoln enjoys watching movies about gangsters from the 1920s who often drink. Lincoln starts drinking here and there with some friends and then begins to binge drink.

   A. Nature or Nurture? _____

   B. List strategies for avoiding alcohol.

   _____

   _____

Name _____ Date _____ Period _____

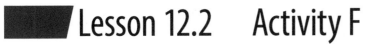 **Lesson 12.2   Activity F**   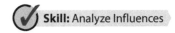 **Skill:** Analyze Influences

Alcohol Ad Analysis

Instructions: *During one evening of watching TV, track the alcohol-related advertisements that you see. Below, record the target audience of the program during which the ad appeared. Also record what alcoholic product each ad was for, and the message or focus of each ad. Then, answer the questions that follow.*

Advertisements

1. Target audience of program: _____

    A. Product advertised: _____

    B. Message/focus of ad: _____

2. Target audience of program: _____

    A. Product advertised: _____

    B. Message/focus of ad: _____

3. Target audience of program: _____

    A. Product advertised: _____

    B. Message/focus of ad: _____

4. Target audience of program: _____

    A. Product advertised: _____

    B. Message/focus of ad: _____

5. Target audience of program: _____

    A. Product advertised: _____

    B. Message/focus of ad: _____

Questions

1. What were the main messages of these alcohol ads?

    _____

    _____

2. If teens saw these ads without knowing anything else about alcohol, what would they think about drinking alcohol? Explain.

    _____

    _____

3. How would you change alcohol-related ads to reduce teen drinking? Explain your reasoning.

    _____

    _____

    _____

    _____

Name _____ Date _____ Period _____

 Lesson 12.2   Activity G

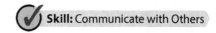

Using Refusal Skills

Instructions: *For each of the following scenarios, explain what you might say to refuse your friend's offer of alcohol. Keep in mind that you may need to leave the situation to avoid further peer pressure. Try to be creative and specific with your responses.*

1. On Saturday evening, you are invited to a party at your friend's house. You decide to go to the party for a few hours. When you arrive, you realize that there are no adults present at the party and that several people have brought alcohol. You are already uncomfortable with the situation, when your friend offers you a drink.

   A. How would you respond?

   _____

   _____

   _____

2. You and a group of friends are hanging out on a Wednesday night. Halfway through the evening, some of your friends decide to start drinking. You know that it is a school night, you have a test first thing in the morning, and you have to leave soon anyway. You're about to leave when your crush offers you a drink and begs you to stay.

   A. How would you respond?

   _____

   _____

   _____

3. On the Friday afternoon before summer vacation starts, you notice invitations to a party being handed out. One of these invitations is slipped into your locker. When you see who is throwing the party, you know that there will be alcohol there. You have made the choice not to drink and you know that people at the party will try to pressure you into drinking.

   A. How would you respond?

   _____

   _____

   _____

4. You and your friends are holding a game night. Everyone is having fun, and you are enjoying just hanging out with your friends and playing games. Someone suggests making the next game a drinking game. Your friends agree and seem to like the idea. They tell you, "it'll be fun," but you were already having fun without alcohol.

   A. How would you respond?

   _____

   _____

   _____

5. You are at a weekend party with alcohol. So far, you have found it easy to refuse your friends' offers of alcohol. Then you notice that the person you have a crush on is also drinking. You really want to impress your crush and have this person like you, but you also do not want to drink. Your crush offers to get you a drink.

   A. How would you respond?

   _____

   _____

Chapter 12   Activity H

Practice Test

Completion

Instructions: *Write the term that completes the statement in the space provided.*

1. _____ is an addictive drug that alters brain function and has substantial effects on the body and a person's thinking and behavior.

   _____

2. The psychological restraint that keeps people from acting in dangerous ways is known as _____.

   _____

3. The condition known as _____ is a buildup of scar tissue in the liver.

   _____

4. Under _____ laws, the only acceptable BAC level for people younger than 21 years of age is 0%.

   _____

5. One of the first steps in treating an alcohol use disorder is a clearing out process known as _____.

   _____

True/False

Instructions: *Indicate whether each statement below is true or false.*

6. _____ *True or false?* Moderate drinking is also known as *social drinking.*

7. _____ *True or false?* Alcohol use can cause strained relationships among family and friends.

8. _____ *True or false?* People who have been drinking alcohol are less likely to behave violently than people who have not.

9. _____ *True or false?* If one twin has an alcohol use disorder, this person's identical twin has no higher likelihood of having an alcohol use disorder.

10. _____ *True or false?* Surrounding yourself with friends who encourage and support your healthy decisions can help you avoid pressure to drink alcohol.

Multiple Choice

Instructions: *Select the letter that corresponds to the correct answer.*

11. _____ Alcohol disrupts functioning of the _____, which controls movement and balance.
    A. medulla
    B. cerebellum
    C. cerebral cortex
    D. pituitary gland

12. _____ Which of the following is *not* a sign of alcohol poisoning?
    A. mental confusion
    B. vomiting
    C. hair loss
    D. hypothermia

13. _____ Which of the following is *not* an environmental factor for alcohol use?
    A. presence of alcohol at family parties
    B. a biological parent with an alcohol use disorder
    C. peer pressure from friends
    D. TV and movies that include alcohol use

14. _____ Self-management techniques for people with alcohol use disorders do *not* include _____.
    A. avoiding situations where alcohol is present
    B. developing strategies for refusing alcohol
    C. engaging in social drinking
    D. learning new strategies for managing stress

Matching

Instructions: *Match each key term to its definition (15–22).*

15. _____ negative symptoms caused by excessive alcohol use

16. _____ operating a motor vehicle with a blood alcohol concentration at or over 0.08% for adults

17. _____ set of health conditions that affect the baby born to a person who has consumed alcohol during the pregnancy

18. _____ medical emergency in which a person consumes more alcohol than the body can break down

19. _____ substance that slows the central nervous system, including the brain

20. _____ substance use disorder in which a person has an addiction to alcohol and continues to consume it despite negative health effects

21. _____ process that allows the body to clear itself of all alcohol or drugs

22. _____ protecting a person from the negative consequences of chosen behaviors

A. alcohol poisoning

B. alcohol use disorder (AUD)

C. depressant

D. detoxification

E. driving under the influence (DUI)

F. enabling

G. fetal alcohol spectrum disorders (FASD)

H. hangover

Analyzing Data

Instructions: *The chart below shows the percentage of high school students who reported drinking alcohol in the past 30 days. This data comes from the Youth Risk Behavior Survey by the CDC. Study the data and answer the questions that follow.*

Percentage of High School Students Who Used Alcohol, by Selected Characteristics									
Characteristic	Total	Male	Female	9th Grade	10th Grade	11th Grade	12th Grade	White Ethnicity	Black Ethnicity	Hispanic Ethnicity
Drinking*	32.8	32.2	33.5	23.4	29	38	42.4	35.2	23.8	34.4
Binge drinking**	17.7	18.6	16.8	10.4	15.1	22.1	24.6	19.7	11.4	17.7

*Had one or more drinks of alcohol during the 30 days before the survey.

**Had five or more drinks in a row (within a couple of hours) during the 30 days before the survey.

Centers for Disease Control and Prevention

Figure 1. Percentage of high school students who used alcohol by biological sex, high school grade, and race/ethnicity

23. What percentage of male teens reported binge drinking? of female teens?

_____

24. What is the difference between the rate at which 10th graders reported drinking and the rate at which they reported binge drinking?

_____

25. Generally, who binge drinks more often—students who identify as white, black, or Hispanic?

_____

Short Answer

Instructions: *Answer the following questions using what you have learned in this chapter.*

26. What do you think is the most persuasive argument that could be used to get teens to stop drinking?

_____

_____

27. If you see a friend or family member abusing alcohol, what is the best thing you can do to help him or her?

_____

_____

Medications and Drugs

Lesson 13.1   Activity A

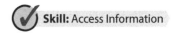 **Skill:** Access Information

Reading Medication Labels

Instructions: *Examine the following label for an over-the-counter cold and flu medication. Answer the following questions related to the label.*

Drug Facts

Active ingredient (in each caplet)   Purpose
Acetaminophen 325 mg . . . . Pain reliever/fever reducer
Dextromethorphan HBr 10 mg . . . . Cough suppressant
Guaifenesin 200 mg . . . . Expectorant
Phenylephrine HCl 5 mg . . . . Nasal decongestant

Uses for the temporary relief of the following cold/flu symptoms:
■ minor aches and pains
■ sore throat
■ cough
■ headache and fever
■ nasal congestion

Warnings
Liver warning
This product contains acetaminophen. The maximum daily dose of this product is 10 caplets (3,250 mg acetaminophen) in 24 hours. Severe liver damage may occur if you take:
■ more than 4,000 mg of acetaminophen in 24 hours
■ with other drugs containing acetaminophen
■ 3 or more alcoholic drinks every day while using this product

Allergy alert
Acetaminophen may cause severe skin reactions. Symptoms may include:
■ skin reddening
■ blisters
■ rash

Sore throat warning
If sore throat is severe, persists for more than 2 days, is accompanied or followed by fever, headache, rash, nausea, or vomiting, consult a doctor promptly.

Drug Facts (continued)

Ask a doctor before use if you are taking blood thinners
Ask a doctor before use if you have
■ liver disease   ■ diabetes
■ heart disease   ■ trouble urinating
■ high blood pressure   ■ persistent or chronic cough
■ thyroid disease

When using this product do not exceed recommended dose
Stop use and ask a doctor if
■ nervousness, dizziness, or sleeplessness occur
■ pain, nasal congestion, or cough gets worse or lasts more than 7 days
■ fever gets worse or lasts more than 3 days
■ redness or swelling is present
■ new symptoms occur
■ cough comes back or occurs with rash or headache that lasts

If pregnant or breast-feeding, ask a health professional before use.
Keep out of reach of children. In case of overdose, get medical help or contact a Poison Control Center right away.

Directions
Adults and children 12 years and over	Take 2 tablets every 4 hours; not more than 10 tablets in 24 hours
Children under 12 years	Ask a doctor

Other information Store at 20–25°C (68–77°F)
■ Do not use if carton is open or broken

Inactive ingredients D&C yellow no. 10, sucralose, magnesium stearate, microcrystalline cellulose, pregelatinized starch

US Department of Health and Human Services

Figure 1. Drug Facts label

1. Why would someone need to take this medication?

_____

_____

2. Based on your age, how much of this medication should you take?

_____

3. What are the health risks of taking this medication?

_____

_____

_____

_____

4. When should you stop using this medication and call a doctor?

_____

_____

_____

_____

_____

5. In which situations should you ask a doctor before using this medication?

_____

_____

_____

_____

_____

6. At what temperature should you store this medication?

_____

7. Do additional research to learn more about the harmful effects of excessive acetaminophen use. Summarize your findings.

_____

_____

_____

_____

_____

_____

_____

_____

_____

_____

_____

_____

8. Provide the citation for your reliable resource.

_____

_____

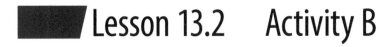 Lesson 13.2   Activity B

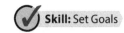

Medication Misuse and Your Goals

Instructions: *Your friend Amelia feels anxious a lot. She has to work hard to stay calm at school, surrounded by so much chaos. Amelia also tosses and turns at night with worry. Yesterday, Amelia texted you "Do you think I should try sedatives? They're supposed to chill people out and help them sleep. It couldn't hurt, right?" Answer the following questions about how misusing depressants can prevent Amelia from achieving her goals.*

1. What does Amelia want to achieve? What is the healthiest way for Amelia to achieve this?

   _____

   _____

2. What are the potential side effects for Amelia of misusing depressants?

   A. Health effects: _____

   _____

   _____

   B. Mental changes: _____

   _____

   _____

   C. Social consequences: _____

   _____

   _____

   D. Legal consequences: _____

   _____

   _____

3. How can depressants become an obstacle that would keep Amelia from reaching her goal from #1? Explain the dangers of self-medicating with medications and drugs.

   _____

   _____

   _____

4. Set a SMART goal to help Amelia overcome the temptation to misuse medications. Whom can she reach out to for help or support? What strategies can she use to improve her health?

   _____

   _____

   _____

   _____

   _____

   _____

   _____

   _____

Lesson 13.2   Activity C

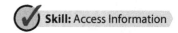

Performance-Enhancing Drugs and Athletes

Instructions: *Some athletes use performance-enhancing drugs (PEDs) to strengthen and increase the size of their muscles and to give themselves a competitive edge. Find a news article about an athlete who used performance-enhancing drugs. Then, answer the questions.*

1. Title of news article: _____

    A. Author(s): _____

    B. Sponsor/organization: _____

2. Who is the athlete who used PEDs?

    _____

3. With which sport and sports organization was this person associated at the time?

    _____

    _____

4. How was the athlete "caught"?

    _____

    _____

    _____

5. Was the athlete punished or penalized for use of PEDs? If so, how?

    _____

    _____

    _____

6. How did being known for having used PEDs impact the person's reputation and career?

    _____

    _____

    _____

    _____

    _____

7. What are possible health consequences of using PEDs?

    _____

    _____

    _____

    _____

    _____

    _____

    _____

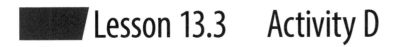 ## Lesson 13.3   Activity D

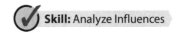

Marijuana Myths

Instructions: *Read the following scenario and answer the questions that follow about the myths teens may hear about marijuana use.*

At 16 years old, this is what Ruth knows about marijuana: Marijuana is dried-up parts of a plant called cannabis. Unlike other illegal drugs, marijuana does not have negative health consequences and is not addictive. If people can use medical marijuana, then it must be safe for everyone to use. When people use marijuana, they do not experience side effects like when they drink alcohol, so they are safe to drive. She would not get into trouble for using marijuana since it is legal in her state. People can use marijuana in lots of ways including blunts, joints, bowls, bongs, vapes, and edibles. Eating a marijuana edible is safer than smoking marijuana.

1. Identify two things that Ruth believes about marijuana that are facts.

   A. Fact: _____

   B. Fact: _____

2. Identify three things that Ruth believes about marijuana that are myths.

   A. Myth: _____

   B. Myth: _____

   C. Myth: _____

3. How can believing these myths influence Ruth's decision-making about marijuana?

   _____

   _____

4. What is the truth behind each myth that Ruth believes? Do additional research as needed.

   A. Myth #1: _____

   _____

   _____

   B. Myth #2: _____

   _____

   _____

   C. Myth #3: _____

   _____

   _____

5. How might knowing the truth behind myths about marijuana use influence Ruth's choices?

   _____

   _____

   _____

   _____

   _____

   _____

Name _____ Date _____ Period _____

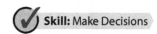

Can This Friendship Be Saved?

Instructions: *David and Jay quickly became friends when they joined the comedy circuit a year ago. They frequently perform in comedy clubs where liquor and drugs are readily available. Jay avoids drugs since he lost an uncle to drug overdose, but David uses a variety of drugs. For each of the following situations, describe what you think Jay should do. Then, explain why you think their friendship can or cannot be saved.*

Situation 1

Each night before he goes onstage to perform, David snorts cocaine. Almost instantly, he feels energetic and mentally alert. Jay thinks that David gets "too wired" because his movements are frantic and the timing for his jokes is off. David tells Jay that the "blow" helps him get through late nights when he worked all day at the TV station.

1. What should Jay say or do?

_____

Situation 2

One night after performing, David's heart is beating so rapidly that he thinks he might be having a heart attack. In addition, David is certain that a new comedian has been "stealing" his jokes and threatens to start a fight. Jay attempts to get David to leave the comedy club and offers to give him a ride home, but David's hostility and paranoia seem unstoppable.

1. What should Jay say or do?

_____

Situation 3

Since David began using drugs, he constantly asks Jay if he can "borrow twenty dollars" for gas or groceries. At first, Jay happily lent his friend the cash. Lately, however, Jay feels like David is taking advantage of him.

1. What should Jay say or do?

_____

Situation 4

One night, David invites Jay and some other comedians to his apartment for some "big H." This is the first time that Jay has heard David mention heroin. Worried for David's safety, Jay reluctantly goes to David's apartment.

1. What should Jay say or do?

_____

2. Based on the situations above, summarize the ways in which David's abuse of illegal drugs affects his friendship with Jay. Do you think the comedians can or should maintain a friendship? Why or why not?

_____

_____

_____

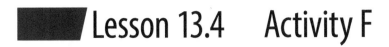 Lesson 13.4   Activity F

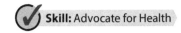 **Skill:** Advocate for Health

Create an Antidrug Advertisement

Instructions: *In small groups, create an antidrug advertisement to convince people to stop or never start abusing drugs (or using illegal drugs). Follow the instructions to get started. Then create your advertisement, using the medium of your choice, and share it with the class. All of the advertisements created by the class will constitute an antidrug campaign.*

Choose a target group.

1. Advertisements are created to appeal to a particular audience. Which group(s) of people will your antidrug advertisement target? Describe your target audience.

   _____

   _____

Choose a focus.

1. Choose an antidrug message you want to communicate. "Using drugs is bad" is too broad a statement. Choose a narrower focus. Consider what kind of antidrug message will appeal to the group you have chosen. Summarize the message of your advertisement in one or two sentences.

   _____

   _____

   _____

   _____

Choose a medium for your message.

1. Choose a medium for your advertisement. Your group might create a flyer, poster, video, podcast, or website. When choosing your medium, consider which medium will best reach your target audience. Describe which medium your group chose and why you chose it.

   _____

   _____

   _____

Create the advertisement.

1. In your groups, create an antidrug advertisement using your chosen medium. Keep your focus and target group in mind as you create. When you have finished, reflect on what you think worked well for your advertisement and what could have worked better.

   _____

   _____

   _____

   _____

   _____

   _____

Lesson 13.4   Activity G

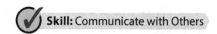 **Skill:** Communicate with Others

Refusal Skills

Instructions: *With a partner, read the following scenarios and brainstorm what you might say to resist using drugs. Use a variety of refusal skills in your responses. Have each partner write down a potential refusal for each scenario and take turns role-playing the situations.*

1. You were part of the school musical that opened tonight and were invited to the cast party at an older student's house. You have heard stories about the drinking and drugs at these parties, and you worry about things getting out of hand. You say as much to your friend, who says, "Oh, don't be a wimp. It's just a party."

   A What would you say?

   _____
   _____
   _____
   _____

2. You have been best friends with Mikko since you were kids, and you trust her. She recently started doing various drugs with her teammates from track, and she invited you to hang out and experiment with them. You express your concern about the drugs, but Mikko says, "I'll take care of you. Don't I always?"

   A What would you say?

   _____
   _____
   _____
   _____

3. Lately, a popular classmate, Nathan, has started interacting with you more at school and online. You hope that being friends with Nathan will help you make more friends. In the busy hallway after school, Nathan asks if you want to buy some ecstasy. When you hesitate, he laughs loudly and says, "Aww man, I was hoping you were *fun*!"

   A What would you say?

   _____
   _____
   _____
   _____

4. You can smell the weed on your older brother, Adam, when he comes home some nights. When you start to ask him about the consequences of smoking weed, Adam cuts you off and explains, "Other drugs are dangerous. Weed isn't that bad; that's why they're legalizing it in so many states!" He then asks if you want to try it with him.

   A What would you say?

   _____
   _____
   _____
   _____

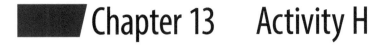 Chapter 13 Activity H

Practice Test

Completion

Instructions: *Write the term that completes the statement in the space provided.*

1. _____ medications are sold to people without a prescription from a doctor or other licensed healthcare professional.

   _____

2. Aspirin, acetaminophen, and ibuprofen are examples of _____, or pain relievers.

   _____

3. All medications can have _____, or unintended changes that develop in response to a medication.

   _____

4. Medication _____ is the use of a medication in an unintended way.

   _____

5. Medication _____ is a persistent pattern of medication misuse that causes harm.

   _____

True/False

Instructions: *Indicate whether each statement below is true or false.*

6. _____ *True or false?* Over-the-counter medications intended for adults can always be given to infants and children.

7. _____ *True or false?* Depressants reduce anxiety and increase a person's ability to relax, stay calm, or sleep.

8. _____ *True or false?* Opioids are typically prescribed to relieve severe, chronic itching.

9. _____ *True or false?* Stimulants are commonly prescribed for people with ADHD.

10. _____ *True or false?* Experts believe that people's genes account for about 50 percent of their risk of developing an addiction.

Multiple Choice

Instructions: *Select the letter that corresponds to the correct answer.*

11. _____ The Food and Drug Administration (FDA) ensures that medications are _____, effective, and secure from tampering.
    A safe to use
    B. approved for in-flight transit
    C delivered to pharmacies quickly
    D kept in a cool, dark location until they are used

12. _____ Some people illegally acquire _____, which they use to gain strength and increase their muscle size.
    A performance-enhancing drugs
    B. stimulants
    C diet pills
    D opioids

13. _____ A chemical called _____ is the active ingredient in marijuana.
    A opium
    B. lysergic acid diethylamide
    C delta-9-tetrahydrocannabinol (THC)
    D cannabis

14. _____ _____ are drugs that can cause a person to see, hear, or feel experiences that are not real.
    A Opioids
    B. Performance-enhancing drugs
    C Bath salts
    D Hallucinogens

15. _____ Which of the following would *not* be an effective strategy for refusing drugs?
    A Provide background for your refusal.
    B. Say "no" without making eye contact.
    C Give an excuse.
    D Change the subject.

Matching

Instructions: *Match each key term to its definition (16–21).*

16. _____ intense pleasurable feeling

17. _____ abuse medications or drugs to cope with symptoms of a health condition

18. _____ act of taking a substance again after deciding to stop

19. _____ the act of consuming addictive, illegal substances

20. _____ increased likelihood of developing negative side effects in response to a particular substance

21. _____ act of taking more of a substance than the body can break down at one time

A drug abuse

B. drug sensitivity

C euphoria

D overdose

E relapse

F. self-medicate

Analyzing Data

Instructions: *Read the data on global opioid use from the United Nations Office on Drugs and Crime to answer the following questions.*

Selected Regions	North America	Asia	Africa	Europe	South America	Global
Number of people using opioids, 2017	12,830,000	29,460,000	6,080,000	3,570,000	580,000	**53,350,000**
Percentage of regional population	3.96	0.98	0.87	0.66	0.20	**1.08**

United Nations Office on Drugs and Crime

Figure 2. Global opioid use

22. What percentage of all of opioid use in the world comes from North America?

_____

23. How many more people use opioids in Asia than in Europe?

_____

Short Answer

Instructions: *Answer the following questions using what you have learned in this chapter.*

24. Explain how taking care of mental health can help prevent medication and drug abuse.

_____

_____

_____

25. Name three treatment programs available for people with substance use disorders.

_____

_____

_____

<table>
</table>

CHAPTER 14

Maintaining Healthy Relationships

Lesson 14.1   Activity A

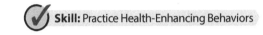 **Skill:** Practice Health-Enhancing Behaviors

Evaluating Relationships

Instructions: *Read each scenario and identify characteristics of the relationship that are healthy and unhealthy. Then, explain how the relationship could be healthier.*

1. Tonya thinks that her next-door neighbor's friends are controlling and disrespectful. She trusts Emilio's judgment, but worries he will get hurt. Tonya wants to tell Emilio her concerns, but worries he will think she is acting jealous.

   A. Identify signs of a healthy or unhealthy relationship.

   _____

   _____

   B. How could the relationship be healthier?

   _____

2. Isabella and Drake work together. They normally have lots of fun together, but Drake tends to yell when he gets irritated. Isabella wishes he would express his frustration in a healthier way, but she does not know how to tell him this.

   A. Identify signs of a healthy or unhealthy relationship.

   _____

   _____

   B. How could the relationship be healthier?

   _____

3. Aspen and his sister, Anna, argue all the time. At the end of the day, though, Aspen knows Anna will always be there for him. Aspen was always a star athlete until high school. Anna helped him come up with a new training program.

   A. Identify signs of a healthy or unhealthy relationship.

   _____

   _____

   B. How could the relationship be healthier?

   _____

4. Malcolm and Daisy have been very happily dating for two years. Malcolm stated his boundaries early on, but lately Daisy has been pressuring him to change these boundaries. Daisy reassures him that he is safe and loved.

   A. Identify signs of a healthy or unhealthy relationship.

   _____

   _____

   B. How could the relationship be healthier?

   _____

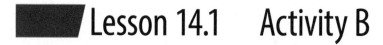 ## Lesson 14.1   Activity B

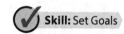

Relationship Goals

Instructions: *Set a SMART goal to improve the quality of your relationships. Answer the following questions to help you achieve your objective.*

1. Create a central goal to improve the quality of your relationships.

_____

_____

2. To be sure your goal is SMART, indicate how it meets each of the following.

    A. Specific: _____

    B. Measurable: _____

    C. Achievable: _____

    D. Relevant: _____

    E. Timely: _____

3. List three short-term goals that will help you achieve your larger goal.

    A. Goal: _____

    _____

    B. Goal: _____

    _____

    C. Goal: _____

    _____

4. Name one obstacle that might stop you from achieving your goal. How can you overcome this obstacle?

_____

_____

_____

_____

_____

5. Whom can you reach out to for help or support in going after your goal?

_____

_____

_____

_____

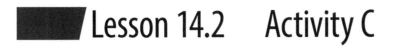 # Lesson 14.2   Activity C

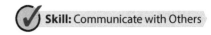 **Skill:** Communicate with Others

Resolving Family Conflicts

Instructions: *The following scenarios describe conflicts between teens and members of their families. After reading each scenario, offer each teen your advice for resolving the conflict. Use the strategies discussed in Lesson 14.2.*

Scenario 1

Drew and his younger brother, Mike, are only a year apart. Last month, Mike got his driver's license and now he wants to use the car all the time. The two brothers are constantly fighting over who gets to drive the car. Since he is the oldest, Drew thinks he should be able to use the car more often than Mike. Their parents are sick of the fighting and have threatened to take the car away from both of them.

1. What advice would you give Drew and Mike about resolving their conflict?

_____

_____

_____

_____

_____

_____

_____

_____

_____

_____

Scenario 2

Olivia's younger sister, Chloe, has been getting on her nerves lately. Chloe comes into Olivia's room without knocking and she keeps wearing Olivia's clothes without asking. Yesterday, Olivia wanted to wear her favorite sweater, but she could not because Chloe had worn it and spilled spaghetti sauce all down the front.

1. What advice would you give Olivia and Chloe about resolving their conflict?

_____

_____

_____

_____

_____

_____

_____

_____

_____

_____

Scenario 3

Isaac is pushing his parents to give him a later curfew. He has to be home by 10:00 p.m. on weekends, but all of his friends stay out until 10:30. Isaac does not understand why his parents will not extend his curfew—especially since it is only by a half hour. Every weekend night he goes out, he feels angry with his parents.

1. What advice would you give Isaac and his parents about resolving their conflict?

_____

_____

_____

_____

_____

_____

_____

_____

_____

Scenario 4

Yvette's grandparents always tell her to put her cell phone away at the dinner table. Yvette cannot understand why they get so upset—it does not take her long to send a text message or two between bites. It seems like she is always fighting with her grandparents about how much time she spends on her phone. Sometimes her grandparents even take her phone away.

1. What advice would you give Yvette and her grandparents about resolving their conflict?

_____

_____

_____

_____

_____

_____

_____

_____

_____

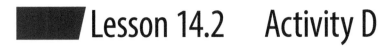 Lesson 14.2 Activity D 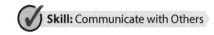 ✓ **Skill:** Communicate with Others

Family Rules

Instructions: *Imagine that your family wants to implement the following family rules and you disagree with them. From the 10 options, choose six family rules about which you feel strongly. Explain why you think these six rules should change. Then, answer the question that follows.*

Family Rules

1. No streaming TV shows during the school week.
   A. Explain why you think the rule should change.

   _____

   _____

   _____

2. No dating before 16 years of age.
   A. Explain why you think the rule should change.

   _____

   _____

   _____

3. No locking your bedroom door.
   A. Explain why you think the rule should change.

   _____

   _____

   _____

4. No phones at the table during dinner.
   A. Explain why you think the rule should change.

   _____

   _____

   _____

5. You must help prepare or clean up after meals.
   A. Explain why you think the rule should change.

   _____

   _____

   _____

6. Curfew on weekends is 10 p.m. sharp.
   A. Explain why you think the rule should change.

   _____

   _____

   _____

7. Every Friday night is family night.

   A. Explain why you think the rule should change.

   _____

   _____

   _____

8. No sleepovers during the school year.

   A. Explain why you think the rule should change.

   _____

   _____

   _____

9. No phone usage after 8 p.m.

   A. Explain why you think the rule should change.

   _____

   _____

   _____

10. Parents/guardians must always know your location.

    A. Explain why you think the rule should change.

    _____

    _____

    _____

Question

1. How can you be assertive about rules you disagree with while still showing respect to your parent or guardian? Explain.

   _____

   _____

   _____

   _____

Name _____ Date _____ Period _____

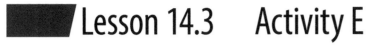 Lesson 14.3   Activity E   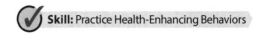 **Skill:** Practice Health-Enhancing Behaviors

Giving Friendship Advice

Instructions: *Imagine you are the first person to welcome Jessica, a new student at your school. For this activity, share with Jessica five tips for making new friends and five strategies for developing healthy friendships. Then, assess your own skills in developing and maintaining healthy friendships.*

1. List five tips for making new friends.

   A. Tip #1: _____

   _____

   B. Tip #2: _____

   _____

   C. Tip #3: _____

   _____

   D. Tip #4: _____

   _____

   E. Tip #5: _____

   _____

2. List five strategies for developing healthy friendships.

   A. Strategy #1: _____

   _____

   B. Strategy #2: _____

   _____

   C. Strategy #3: _____

   _____

   D. Strategy #4: _____

   _____

   E. Strategy #5: _____

   _____

3. Assess your own skills in developing and maintaining healthy friendships. What do you do well? What could you do better?

   _____

   _____

   _____

   _____

   _____

   _____

   _____

Name _____ Date _____ Period _____

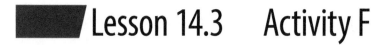 Lesson 14.3   Activity F

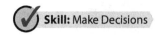

Rewrite the Story

Instructions: *As you read the following scenarios, identify mistakes each teen makes that could interfere with the development of healthy friendships. Then, rewrite the stories by changing these mistakes and adding strategies to build and maintain healthy friendships.*

Scenario 1

> Nikita has a very full schedule. Between school, swim team, and band, Nikita feels like she hardly has enough time to sleep, let alone spend time with friends. She chats with her friends between activities, but feels like she cannot keep up with the group chats. Each night, Nikita eats dinner, watches TV for a few hours, finishes her homework, and is off to bed.

1. What mistakes does Nikita make that may interfere with developing healthy friendships?

   _____

   _____

   _____

2. Rewrite the scenario with additional strategies for building and maintaining healthy friendships.

   _____

   _____

   _____

   _____

   _____

   _____

   _____

Scenario 2

> Joe has always had a difficult time expressing himself. When he notices his friend, Emmanuel, spending time with new friends more than with him, he asks, "So that's how it's gonna be, huh? I'm nothing to you now?" Confused, Emmanuel tries to talk to Joe. Feeling wronged, Joe does not explain himself. Now, Emmanuel spends more time with his other friends than ever.

1. What mistakes does Joe make that may interfere with developing healthy friendships?

   _____

   _____

   _____

2. Rewrite the scenario with additional strategies for building and maintaining healthy friendships.

   _____

   _____

   _____

   _____

   _____

Name _____ Date _____ Period _____

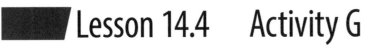 Lesson 14.4   Activity G   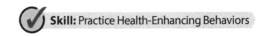 **Skill:** Practice Health-Enhancing Behaviors

Healthy Versus Unhealthy

Instructions: *Answer the reflection question about dating relationships. Then, read the following scenarios about teen dating relationships. Decide whether each couple seems to have a healthy or unhealthy dating relationship, and then explain how this relationship can be healthier.*

1. List at least five qualities you would want in a healthy dating relationship.

_____

_____

_____

_____

_____

Scenario 1

Chris and Hannah have been dating for three months. Hannah really likes Chris, but he has been acting jealous lately. Every day, he asks who she is texting and gets upset if it is one of her male friends. Last week, Hannah's friend, Blake, gave her a ride to the football game, and Chris was so angry he would not speak to her for the rest of the night.

1. Is this dating relationship healthy or unhealthy? _____

2. How can this relationship be healthier?

_____

_____

Scenario 2

Kai and Andy are involved in many activities, but they try to support each other as much as they can. Kai attends as many of Andy's baseball games as her rehearsal schedule allows; and when Kai was the lead in the school play, no one cheered louder for her than Andy. Kai and Andy's friends complain that they only spend time with each other anymore.

1. Is this dating relationship healthy or unhealthy? _____

2. How can this relationship be healthier?

_____

_____

Scenario 3

Each morning, Owen leaves the house early so he can pick up his girlfriend, Katie, on his way to school. He tries to give Katie thoughtful gifts and do nice things for her, such as offering her rides because she does not have a car. Lately, though, Owen has been feeling like he is just Katie's chauffeur. When she forgot his birthday last week, his feelings were really hurt.

1. Is this dating relationship healthy or unhealthy? _____

2. How can this relationship be healthier?

_____

_____

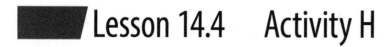 ## Lesson 14.4   Activity H

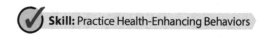

Enforcing Your Boundaries

Instructions: *Imagine that you are in the following scenarios and your boundaries and limits are being threatened. Decide what you would do to enforce these boundaries. Then, answer the reflection question.*

Scenarios

1. You know that your dating partner loves you. You are afraid to express your limits around sexual activity, however, because you do not know how your partner will respond.

   A. What would you do to enforce your boundaries?

   _____

   _____

2. Your dating partner likes to text you late at night. You always want to talk to your partner, but you are exhausted the next day. You are beginning to get upset that your partner does not seem to care if you get enough sleep.

   A. What would you do to enforce your boundaries?

   _____

   _____

3. You have repeatedly communicated to your dating partner that you would like to spend more time with your friends. Your partner continues to get upset when you choose to spend time with other people.

   A. What would you do to enforce your boundaries?

   _____

   _____

Reflection Questions

1. Explain the importance of deciding on and communicating your boundaries early in a relationship.

   _____

   _____

   _____

2. Imagine that you do not enforce your boundaries. How might this affect a dating relationship? How might this affect your health?

   _____

   _____

   _____

   _____

3. What should you do if your dating partner does not respect your boundaries? Explain.

   _____

   _____

   _____

   _____

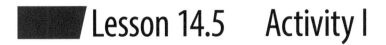 Lesson 14.5   Activity I   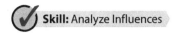 Skill: Analyze Influences

Factors Affecting Abstinence

Instructions: *Read the following scenarios and answer the questions about the influences that may affect Aliah's decision to practice sexual abstinence.*

Scenario 1

Going into high school, all sorts of exciting new things are coming Aliah's way. She finally gets to drive, she has a new job, and she is going on dates. She does not think she is ready for a sexual relationship. She just wants to have fun without it getting that intense.

1. What factors may influence Aliah's decision to practice abstinence?

_____

_____

2. How might this decision be challenged throughout high school? How can Aliah overcome these challenges?

_____

_____

Scenario 2

Aliah has started dating someone and she feels completely comfortable with this person. She enjoys the physical intimacy with this person, but she always stops short of having sex because she does not want to deal with a pregnancy or STI. Even if the risk is small, it is a risk she does not want to have at all.

1. What factors influence Aliah's decision to practice abstinence?

_____

_____

2. What factors may influence Aliah's decision not to practice abstinence? How can she overcome these factors?

_____

_____

Scenario 3

Aliah knows that her best friend and her best friend's dating partner had sex last year and they have never felt closer or more intimate. Aliah fears that not progressing sexually in her relationship means that her relationship is not healthy. When she expresses her fears to her partner, her partner says that sexual compatibility is a big part of a long-term relationship.

1. What factors influence Aliah's decision to practice abstinence?

_____

_____

2. What factors may influence Aliah's decision not to practice abstinence? How can she overcome these factors?

_____

_____

Name _____ Date _____ Period _____

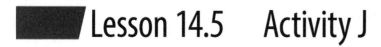 Lesson 14.5   Activity J   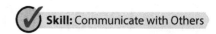 **Skill:** Communicate with Others

Continuous Abstinence

Instructions: *Respond to the following lines pressuring you to have sex by respectfully and assertively saying "no" to sex. Include benefits of abstinence in your response.*

Pressure Lines

1. We have been dating for years and I love you. I want this night to be special for both of us.

    A. Provide a response: _____

    _____

2. Sex isn't that big of a deal. It won't change anything between us.

    A. Provide a response: _____

    _____

3. We love each other, right? And we want to get married one day? Then why wait?

    A. Provide a response: _____

    _____

4. I know you want to try it. Let's just have fun and see what it's like.

    A. Provide a response: _____

    _____

5. I have always been here for you. If you really loved me, you would want to do this with me.

    A. Provide a response: _____

    _____

6. Do you think I would hurt you? I love you and I always will.

    A. Provide a response: _____

    _____

Questions

1. Name at least three situations that may increase your risk of compromising your boundaries about sexual activity.

    _____

    _____

2. Explain how body language can either reinforce or undermine the communication of your boundaries. Provide examples.

    _____

    _____

3. What might you need to do if a dating partner questions, teases, or pressures you about your boundaries? Explain.

    _____

    _____

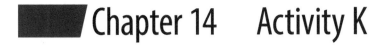 Chapter 14   Activity K

Practice Test

Completion

Instructions: *Write the term that completes the statement in the space provided.*

1. Respecting a person's boundaries includes giving and receiving _____ consent, which is a direct, verbal, freely given agreement.

_____

2. Competing with a sibling for material or nonmaterial items is sibling _____.

_____

3. A(n) _____ is a small group of friends who deliberately exclude other people from joining or being part of their group.

_____

4. Attraction without closeness is called a(n) _____.

_____

5. Feelings of _____ are intense romantic feelings that develop suddenly and are usually based on physical attraction.

_____

True/False

Instructions: *Indicate whether each statement below is true or false.*

6. _____ *True or false?* People with social support are less likely to get sick, recover from disease faster, and live longer than people who lack social support.

7. _____ *True or false?* Your immediate family includes siblings, parents or guardians, aunts, uncles, cousins, and grandparents.

8. _____ *True or false?* Because of the lack of in-person interaction, close friendships cannot develop between online friends.

9. _____ *True or false?* Relationships that are full of stress, tension, and conflict can negatively affect your health.

10. _____ *True or false?* Your individuality becomes less important when you enter a dating relationship.

Multiple Choice

Instructions: *Select the letter that corresponds to the correct answer.*

11. _____ Which of the following is a sign of an unhealthy relationship?
    A. feeling one can never say anything right   C. mocking or making fun of
    B. extreme jealousy   D. All of the above.

12. _____ Which of the following is an effective strategy for managing sibling relationships?
    A. Share your private space together.   C. Do not leave a conflict until it is resolved.
    B. Keep your sibling conflicts to yourselves. D. Compromise on recurring issues.

13. _____ Which of the following types of friendships includes a lack of in-person interaction?
    A. casual friends   C. acquaintances
    B. online friends   D. All of the above.

14. _____ Which of the following describes a typically short-lived attraction based on physical attraction rather than a deeper, longer-lasting emotional connection?
    A. love   C. closeness
    B. exclusivity   D. passion

15. _____ Which of the following is true of sexual abstinence?
    A. decreases risk of STIs and HIV
    B. decreases time for growth in other parts of life
    C. increases pain following a breakup
    D. A and B.

Matching

Instructions: *Match each key term to its definition (16–22).*

16. _____ people who work for the same employer or do the same kind of work

17. _____ hormone released during sexual activity that promotes bonding and connection

18. _____ romantically involved only with a partner

19. _____ spending time in a group that includes someone a person is interested in romantically

20. _____ shared or exhibited by both sides

21. _____ people in a person's social circle who may not be close enough to be friends

22. _____ emotion characterized by wanting or being unhappy about another person's positive experiences or circumstances

A. acquaintances
B. coworkers
C. exclusive
D. group dating
E. jealousy
F. oxytocin
G. reciprocal

Analyzing Data

Instructions: *Read the data provided from the Pew Research Center about households containing two or more adult generations. Then, use that information to answer the following questions.*

Percent of US Population Living in Multigenerational Households						
Year	Total	Asian	African American	Hispanic	Other	Caucasian
2009	17	26	24	23	20	13
2016	20	29	26	27	21	16

Pew Research Center

Figure 1. Number of households containing two or more adult generations by race

23. Which ethnic group is most likely in 2016 to live in a multigenerational household? least likely?

_____

24. What effect does the growing minority population in the US have on the overall rates of living in multigenerational households?

_____

25. What factors do you think may influence the increase in the percentage of people living in multigenerational households?

_____

_____

Short Answer

Instructions: *Answer the following questions using what you have learned in this chapter.*

26. What are three common issues in friendships?

_____

_____

27. Name five characteristics of healthy dating relationships.

_____

_____

_____

Name _____ Date _____ Period _____

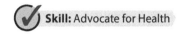

CHAPTER 15 Violence Prevention and Response

Lesson 15.1   Activity A

Skill: Advocate for Health

Be the Friend

Instructions: *Read the following scenarios and decide how you can help someone who is being bullied. Use several different strategies based on the scenarios. Lastly, identify how your influence could positively impact the person being bullied.*

1. Your teammates humiliate Riley in the locker room after practice because Riley is the newest member of the team. You remember what it was like to be the new member.

   A. Describe how you can help.

   _____

   _____

   B. How can your influence positively impact Riley?

   _____

2. In PE class every day, a student touches, hugs, and makes sexual jokes to Clarke. This occurs every class, and it is obvious that Clarke is uncomfortable and embarrassed.

   A. Describe how you can help.

   _____

   _____

   B. How can your influence positively impact Clarke?

   _____

3. Morgan wears dated clothing and some other students spread a rumor that Morgan is homeless. While you have not participated in the gossip, you have done nothing to stop it.

   A. Describe how you can help.

   _____

   _____

   B. How can your influence positively impact Morgan?

   _____

4. You and Reese have lockers next to each other. Most days, an older student knocks Reese's books to the ground. Reese has started to look anxious during every passing period.

   A. Describe how you can help.

   _____

   _____

   B. How can your influence positively impact Reese?

   _____

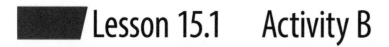 Lesson 15.1   Activity B   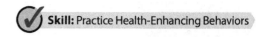 **Skill:** Practice Health-Enhancing Behaviors

Consequences of Cyberbullying

Instructions: *Read the following examples of cyberbullying. Decide how you would respond if you were the person in each situation. Use several different strategies based on the scenarios. Then, answer the question that follows.*

Cyberbullying Examples

1. **Social media post:** Wish Audrey and her people would go back to where they came from and leave my country alone.
   A. How would you respond?

   _____

2. **Group text:** I hate my ex so much. Look at this stupid nude photo he sent me.
   A. How would you respond?

   _____

3. **Social media post:** Anybody else hear that Rafael's mom cheated on his dad? How embarrassing!
   A. How would you respond?

   _____

4. **Group text:** Let's see how much alcohol we can get Miranda to drink before we let her into our group.
   A. How would you respond?

   _____

5. **Social media post:** Like this post if you wish Trey would just disappear.
   A. How would you respond?

   _____

6. **Text message:** You looked hot at practice today. You can't hide from me—I know your whole schedule.
   A. How would you respond?

   _____

7. **Social media post:** Priya is so boring! It's no wonder she has no friends.
   A. How would you respond?

   _____

Question

1. Predict the physical, mental and emotional, and social effects for the people who are cyberbullied.

   _____

   _____

   _____

   _____

   _____

   _____

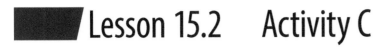 Lesson 15.2   Activity C

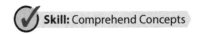 **Skill:** Comprehend Concepts

Importance of Affirmed Consent

Instructions: *Review the information about consent in your textbook. Then read the following scenarios and determine whether consent has been given in each. Explain each answer.*

1. Fifteen-year-old Keisha is excited to be at a party. A student named Brad approaches Keisha, and she is surprised that he wants to talk to her. Brad asks if she wants to have sex. Keisha agrees.

   A. Was consent given? Explain why or why not.

   _____

   _____

2. Both 45 years old, Maria and Cooper have been married for 15 years and have three children. They have had sex many times, so Maria does not ask Cooper for consent this time. She assumes that she has his consent.

   A. Was consent given? Explain why or why not.

   _____

   _____

3. By the time Jensen, who is 26 years old, leaves the bar, he is so intoxicated that he can barely stand. On his way out, Jensen tells his friend Cassie that he likes her dress. Cassie asks him if he would like to have sex, and he mumbles an agreement.

   A. Was consent given? Explain why or why not.

   _____

   _____

4. Max asks his 20-year-old girlfriend Brianna if she wants to have sex. Brianna tells Max that she does not want to have sex. Max makes fun of her, calling her a prude. Feeling embarrassed, Brianna says, "Okay."

   A. Was consent given? Explain why or why not.

   _____

   _____

5. Izzy and Santino met around the time they turned 22. Santino likes Izzy, and he asks him if he wants to have sex with him. Looking him in the eye, he smiles and says, "Yeah, Santino. I do."

   A. Was consent given? Explain why or why not.

   _____

   _____

6. Thirty-year-old Jason has been dating Luna, who is 32, for a few months. Their sexual relationship has been slowly progressing, and Jason asks her if she is ready to have sex. Looking nervous, Luna says, "Ummm… okay. Sure."

   A. Was consent given? Explain why or why not.

   _____

   _____

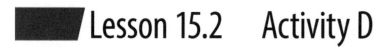 Lesson 15.2   Activity D

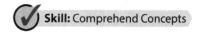 **Skill:** Comprehend Concepts

Sexual Harassment

Instructions: *Read each of the following scenarios and identify whether each action is an example of verbal or nonverbal sexual harassment. Provide a possible response to the situation. Remember that a response can include directly replying to the incident, notifying authority figures after the fact, or even advocating for change in your community. Then, answer the question that follows.*

Scenarios

1. Ethan asks Paloma out on a date every time she walks into the classroom, even though she always says "no."

   A. Verbal or nonverbal? _____

   B. How would you respond? _____

   _____

2. Annie comes up behind Jackson one day during gym class and pulls his shorts to the ground.

   A. Verbal or nonverbal? _____

   B. How would you respond? _____

   _____

3. Zack stares at Kayla's chest any time she tries to have a conversation with him, making her uncomfortable.

   A. Verbal or nonverbal? _____

   B. How would you respond? _____

   _____

4. Aria tells Rodrigo that she loves the way his butt looks in his school pants and that it turns her on.

   A. Verbal or nonverbal? _____

   B. How would you respond? _____

   _____

5. A car drives past Arath and honks the horn. The driver rolls down her window and makes kissing noises at him.

   A. Verbal or nonverbal? _____

   B. How would you respond? _____

   _____

6. Sean brushes against Nina's backside. Nina says something to her about it, and she pinches her thigh and tells her to relax.

   A. Verbal or nonverbal? _____

   B. How would you respond? _____

   _____

Question

1. What are some possible health consequences for a person who experiences sexual harassment?

   _____

   _____

Name _____ Date _____ Period _____

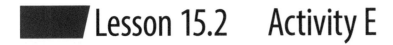 Lesson 15.2   Activity E

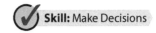

Taking Precautions

Instructions: *Read each of the scenarios presented and identify what each person should do to ensure their safety and avoid experiencing sexual assault.*

Scenario 1

Willa is at a graduation party where everyone is outside in the backyard. She is talking to Kevin, who is very charming and interesting. So far, it seems that they share a lot of interests and hobbies. Willa is enjoying herself until Kevin suddenly says he has to show her something in the kitchen. Willa thinks this is strange, and it seems even stranger when Kevin insists that she put down her drink so he can take her hand and lead her into the kitchen.

1. What decision can Willa make to protect herself from sexual assault?

_____

_____

Scenario 2

Damien and Rosalie are studying for an exam in their health class at Rosalie's house. He has never been here before and her parents are out for the evening. Before Damien and Rosalie have finished their practice test, Rosalie tugs at Damien's shirt and suggests that they take some pictures. She picks up her phone and tells Damien to remove his clothes. "No," he replies, "I don't want pictures of myself like that online." Rosalie insists. Damien is worried she will not take no for an answer.

1. What decision can Damien make to protect himself from sexual assault?

_____

_____

Scenario 3

Ellie is hanging out with some friends and her crush, Jacob. Everyone is getting along well and having a good time. Ellie and Jacob spend a long time chatting with each other. As it gets late, several people begin to arrange carpools to get back home. Jacob offers to drive Ellie home. Ellie appreciates the offer, but she does not know Jacob very well. Although she has had a crush on him for a while, tonight is the first time she has talked to him properly.

1. What decision can Ellie make to protect herself from sexual assault?

_____

_____

Scenario 4

Thursday night, Matthias gets a text message from one of his friends. There is a big party going on the next night and Matthias is invited. Matthias's friend tells him that no adults will be at the party, so it will be extra fun. Matthias's friend also tells him that there will probably be alcohol at the party, so it is best if he does not tell his parents where he is going.

1. What decision can Matthias make to protect himself from sexual assault?

_____

_____

Scenario 5

Chantel and a few of her friends have an important chemistry test coming up. They all meet at the public library after school to study and are there all afternoon and evening. Chantel's friends are picked up by their parents, but Chantel borrowed the family's minivan to drive herself home. Everyone leaves the library when it closes at 9:00 p.m., and Chantel must walk to her car alone in the dark parking lot.

1. What decision can Chantel make to protect herself from sexual assault?

_____

_____

Scenario 6

One night, Mason works the late shift at his part-time job at the grocery store. No one can pick him up this late, so he walks home alone. A car drives up next to him and slows down. The clean-cut person driving the car asks if Mason would like a ride. Mason is tired after his long shift.

1. What decision can Mason make to protect himself from sexual assault?

_____

_____

Scenario 7

Esmeralda loves meeting new people online and chatting with them about her interests. Last month, she started talking with an online friend who shares many of her hobbies. Her online friend recently asked if they could meet in person.

1. What decision can Esmeralda make to protect herself from sexual assault?

_____

_____

Scenario 8

Marcus wants to go to a baseball game with his friends. His mom is working that day so she cannot drive him, and he does not have his driver's license yet. Instead, he orders a car through his mom's account on a rideshare app. He thinks about texting his mom to let her know when he gets in the car and again when he arrives safely, but does not want to bother her at work.

1. What decision can Marcus make to protect himself from sexual assault?

_____

_____

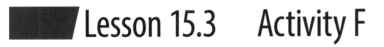 Lesson 15.3   Activity F

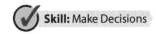 Skill: Make Decisions

Reporting Abuse

Instructions: *Read the following scenarios and identify the type of abuse, the pros and cons of reporting it, and potential consequences of not reporting it for each person.*

Scenario 1

Julie has been dating Asif for two years. Julie has noticed a pattern of unhealthy behaviors from Asif, but knows that Asif was mistreated in the past. He insists that Julie stop talking to her friends because he said they "disrespect" him. Asif drops by uninvited to check up on Julie and wrongfully accuses her of flirting with others. He has even insisted on having access to Julie's phone password and GPS location.

1. What type of abuse is occurring? _____

2. From the perspective of Julie, what are the potential pros and cons of reporting the abuse?

    A. Pros: _____

    _____

    B. Cons: _____

    _____

3. What are the potential consequences for Julie if she does not report the abuse?

    _____

    _____

    _____

    _____

Scenario 2

As twins, Kyle and Davis are very competitive. Both make very good grades and have similar interests. When Kyle gets a better grade than his brother, Davis usually goes home and beats him up. Davis will kick and punch Kyle until he begs him to stop. Kyle's parents tell him that fighting is normal for boys. Kyle has started to fail his classes on purpose because he is afraid of his brother.

1. What type of abuse is occurring? _____

2. From the perspective of Kyle, what are the potential pros and cons of reporting the abuse?

    A. Pros: _____

    _____

    B. Cons: _____

    _____

3. What are the potential consequences for Kyle if he does not report the abuse?

    _____

    _____

    _____

    _____

Scenario 3

Ever since Brandy moved to an assisted living home, she has not been the same. She has withdrawn from family and friends and does not engage in conversation during their visits. Brandy is yelled at and belittled by the caretakers at the assisted living home. They only bring her food and water once a day and rarely help her bathe. She feels helpless in her home.

1. What type of abuse is occurring? _____

2. From the perspective of Brandy, what are the potential pros and cons of reporting the abuse?

    A. Pros: _____

    _____

    B. Cons: _____

    _____

3. What are the potential consequences for Brandy if she does not report the abuse?

_____

_____

_____

_____

Scenario 4

When Gael's dad died at a young age, his mom was overcome with grief. Leaning on alcohol and drugs to cope, she developed a substance use disorder. She was fired from her job, and at 14, Gael cannot yet work. Gael and his mom often do not have enough money for clothes or food. Gael has also been attacked by violent people because his mother owes them money for drugs.

1. What type of abuse is occurring? _____

2. From the perspective of Gael, what are the potential pros and cons of reporting the abuse?

    A. Pros: _____

    _____

    B. Cons: _____

    _____

3. What are the potential consequences for Gael if he does not report the abuse?

_____

_____

_____

_____

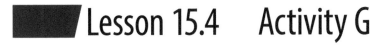 Lesson 15.4   Activity G

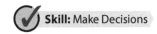 Skill: Make Decisions

What Would You Do?

Instructions: *With a partner, brainstorm three alternative decisions you can make to respond to the violence in each scenario. Then, discuss the pros and cons of each choice. Select the best alternative for each teen and explain your choice.*

Scenario 1

> You learn through the grapevine at school that two of the boys in your class are plotting to "exact revenge" on those who have bullied them. You hear that the boys are planning to bring weapons to school.

1. List three alternatives and the pros and cons of each.

   A. Alternative: _____

      Pros: _____

      _____

      Cons: _____

      _____

   B. Alternative: _____

      Pros: _____

      _____

      Cons: _____

      _____

   C. Alternative: _____

      Pros: _____

      _____

      Cons: _____

      _____

2. Which is the best alternative? Why?

   _____

   _____

Scenario 2

> A new student who is a Muslim has begun to attend your school. Almost immediately, she starts to receive anonymous, threatening letters; and other students routinely make insulting remarks about her religion, cultural clothing, and ethnicity. One afternoon, you witness someone pushing her and tossing her books onto the floor.

1. List three alternatives and the pros and cons of each.

   A. Alternative: _____

      Pros: _____

Cons: _____

_____

B. Alternative: _____

Pros: _____

_____

Cons: _____

_____

C. Alternative: _____

Pros: _____

_____

Cons: _____

_____

2. Which is the best alternative? Why?

_____

_____

Scenario 3

You have made a new friend at school, but the more you get to know your friend, the more her behavior worries you. Your friend is often absent from school and when you ask her about it, she gives a rehearsed-sounding speech about traveling to other cities. When she does attend school, she has bruises in various stages of healing and seems timid.

1. List three alternatives and the pros and cons of each.

A. Alternative: _____

Pros: _____

_____

Cons: _____

_____

B. Alternative: _____

Pros: _____

_____

Cons: _____

_____

C. Alternative: _____

Pros: _____

_____

Cons: _____

_____

2. Which is the best alternative? Why?

_____

_____

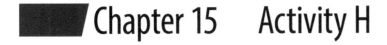 Chapter 15   Activity H

Practice Test

Completion

Instructions: *Write the term that completes the statement in the space provided.*

1. _____ is aggressive behavior toward someone that causes the person injury or discomfort.

   _____

2. When an adult does not meet a child's basic physical, emotional, medical, or educational needs, this is considered _____.

   _____

3. Looking at children or teens sexually, or _____, is a type of child abuse.

   _____

4. _____ abuse is behaviors or neglect that cause harm to someone 60 years of age or older.

   _____

5. Human _____ is a form of modern slavery in which people are forced or pressured to perform a job or service against their will.

   _____

True/False

Instructions: *Indicate whether each statement below is true or false.*

6. _____ *True or false?* Bullying is a physical action; it does not include threatening behavior.

7. _____ *True or false?* Hazing is a type of bullying that uses group pressure to make someone do embarrassing or dangerous activity to be accepted into a group.

8. _____ *True or false?* Sometimes the people who experience sexual assault are to blame.

9. _____ *True or false?* Consent is when someone does not say "no" to sexual activity.

10. _____ *True or false?* Intimate partner violence occurs only between married couples.

Multiple Choice

Instructions: *Select the letter that corresponds to the correct answer.*

11. _____ Which of the following describes social bullying?
    A. mocking someone's religious beliefs
    B. humiliating the new members of your team
    C. ignoring a person who sits with you at lunch
    D. B and C.

12. _____ Which of the following examples of sexual harassment would be considered nonverbal?
    A. catcalling whistles or kissing noises
    B. making sexual jokes
    C. spreading sexual rumors
    D. asking sexual questions

13. _____ Attitudes, controlling behaviors, or words that harm a person's mental health is _____ abuse.
    A. physical
    B. emotional
    C. sexual
    D. financial

14. _____ School violence includes any violent behavior that occurs _____.
    A. on school property
    B. at school-sponsored events
    C. on the way to or from school or school events
    D. All of the above.

Matching

Instructions: *Match each key term to its definition (15–20).*

15. _____ individual required by law to report signs of abuse

16. _____ any kind of violence or threat of violence that targets people because of their race, ethnicity, disability, or religion

17. _____ sexual intercourse between an adult and anyone under the age of consent

18. _____ act of pretending to be someone else online

19. _____ person who is present at a situation, but does not participate or intervene

20. _____ following and repeatedly contacting someone using electronic communication, causing the person to feel scared, nervous, or threatened

A. bystander

B. cyberstalking

C. hate crime

D. impersonation

E. mandated reporter

F. statutory rape

Analyzing Data

Instructions: *Read the data from the Pew Research Center to answer the following questions.*

Percent of US Teens Who Have Experienced Cyberbullying			
Type of Cyberbullying	Total	Female	Male
Offensive name-calling	42%	42%	41%
Spreading of false rumors	32%	39%	26%
Receiving explicit images they did not ask for	25%	29%	20%
Constant asking of where they are, what they're doing, who they're with, by someone other than a parent or guardian	21%	23%	18%
Physical threats	16%	16%	16%
Having explicit images of them shared without their consent	7%	9%	5%
Any type of cyberbullying listed above	59%	60%	59%

Pew Research Center

Figure 1. Types of cyberbullying experienced by teens

21. Using the rates from this survey, how many teens at your school have experienced cyberbullying of any type?

_____

22. Why do you think females experience certain types of cyberbullying, like spreading rumors or nonconsensual explicit images, at a higher rate than males?

_____

_____

Short Answer

Instructions: *Answer the following question using what you have learned in this chapter.*

23. List three potential risk factors and three protective factors for abuse.

_____

_____

_____

_____

_____

_____

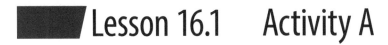

CHAPTER 16 / Personal Safety

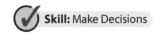

Skill: Make Decisions

Lesson 16.1   Activity A

What Would You Do?

Instructions: *Read the following scenarios and decide what you would do in each situation. Then, explain how future incidents can be prevented.*

1. Your sister drives you to and from school, and one day, she is tired because she hardly got any sleep. Suddenly, the car veers into oncoming traffic. You yell and your sister wakes up in time to pull the car back into the correct lane.

   A. What would you do?

   _____

   _____

   _____

   B. How can future incidents be prevented?

   _____

   _____

2. After school, you and your friend wander around waiting for your dad to pick you both up. You walk under the bleachers in the gym, and your friend asks, "Hey, what is that?" Your friend points to a bag on the ground. In the bag, you find a gun.

   A. What would you do?

   _____

   _____

   _____

   B. How can future incidents be prevented?

   _____

   _____

3. Your mom starts the car in the attached garage in the morning so it can heat up before you leave. The smoke and carbon monoxide detectors are on your kitchen counter because they need new batteries.

   A. What would you do?

   _____

   _____

   _____

   B. How can future incidents be prevented?

   _____

   _____

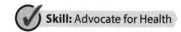

Lesson 16.1   Activity B

Skill: Advocate for Health

Safety on the Road

Instructions: *Set a SMART goal to maintain road safety. Fill in the following information to help you achieve your objective.*

1. Explain the importance of practicing safety strategies as a pedestrian, driver, and passenger.

   _____

   _____

   _____

2. Create a central goal to stay safe on the road.

   _____

   _____

   _____

3. To be sure your goal is SMART, indicate how it meets each of the following.

   A. Specific: _____

   B. Measurable: _____

   C. Achievable: _____

   D. Relevant: _____

   E. Timely: _____

4. List three short-term goals that will help you achieve your larger goal.

   A. Goal: _____

   _____

   _____

   B. Goal: _____

   _____

   _____

   C. Goal: _____

   _____

   _____

5. Name one obstacle that might stop you from achieving your goal. How can you overcome this obstacle?

   _____

   _____

   _____

   _____

   _____

   _____

   _____

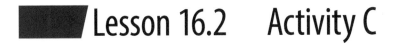 Lesson 16.2   Activity C

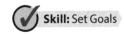

Staying Safe Home Alone

Instructions: *Read the following scenarios about safety when home alone. From the teen's perspective in each scenario, consider the pros and cons of each decision. Based on the information presented in Lesson 16.2, decide on the safest decision to make. Defend your answer.*

Scenario 1

While doing her homework after school, Charlize's doorbell rings. Her parents do not get home from work for another hour. Peeking through the window, she sees a delivery person with a box. Charlize remembers that something her parents ordered was due to arrive this week. Charlize moves to unlock the door.

1. What are the pros and cons of Charlize unlocking and opening her door?

   A. Pros: _____

   _____

   B. Cons: _____

   _____

2. Should Charlize open the door for a stranger when she is home alone? Defend your answer.

   _____

   _____

   _____

   _____

Scenario 2

Elian loves how connected social media makes him feel to his friends and dating partner, who goes to another school. Home alone, he posts a series of pictures playing with his dog, making dinner, and doing homework. Getting ready for bed, Elian writes, "Another night alone. Guess I'll just tuck myself in." Before posting it, however, he hesitates.

1. What are the pros and cons of Elian posting this message?

   A. Pros: _____

   _____

   B. Cons: _____

   _____

2. Should Elian post his message? Defend your answer.

   _____

   _____

   _____

   _____

Scenario 3

Hayden gets home from school and miraculously does not have any homework or studying to do. No one is home to hang out with him, so Hayden texts his neighbor, who is also not busy. They decide to go to the park to play catch. Hayden is going to leave his phone at home, and wonders if he should call his parents first to tell them where he is going.

1. What are the pros and cons of Hayden calling his parents?

   A. Pros: _____

   _____

   B. Cons: _____

   _____

2. Should Hayden call his parents? Defend your answer.

   _____

   _____

   _____

   _____

Scenario 4

Emma is having a hard time with the new section in her chemistry homework. She would ask her mom for help, but she works late tonight, so Emma is home alone. Emma messages her lab partner, who she did not know before this class. Her lab partner offers to come over and help her with the homework.

1. What are the pros and cons of Emma inviting her lab partner over?

   A. Pros: _____

   _____

   B. Cons: _____

   _____

2. Should Emma invite her lab partner over? Defend your answer.

   _____

   _____

   _____

   _____

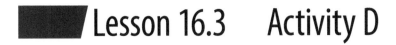 Lesson 16.3 Activity D

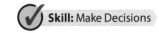

Addressing Risky Situations

Instructions: *Read the following scenarios and write a response that would help maintain the safety of each teen. Use the communication skills you learned in Chapter 3.*

1. Brie and Alani met about a year ago through the video game they both play. They have so much in common and are both the same age. One day, Alani texts Brie, "Wanna meet up this weekend?"

    A. Write your response.

    _____

    _____

    _____

    _____

    _____

    _____

    _____

    _____

2. Nick and his friends love finding new music and sharing it with one another. One day, Nick's friend sends him a strange link and says, "Check out this leaked song I found!"

    A. Write your response.

    _____

    _____

    _____

    _____

    _____

    _____

    _____

    _____

3. Emory was looking through the comments on a social media post for her favorite comedian. Someone commented "YOU AREN'T EVEN FUNNY!!!! GET A REAL JOB."

    A. Write your response.

    _____

    _____

    _____

    _____

    _____

    _____

    _____

4. Leon made his social media profiles public. One day, he posts a selfie saying, "Hanging at school for a few hours until my ride gets here. Ask me questions!"

A. Write your response.

_____

_____

_____

_____

_____

_____

_____

_____

5. Lucy has been saving up her money to buy a new tablet for her artwork. One day, Lucy gets an email that says, "Win a free tablet today! Click on the link here."

A. Write your response.

_____

_____

_____

_____

_____

_____

_____

_____

6. Darren's dating partner sometimes sends sexually explicit messages that make him uncomfortable. Darren just received this text from his partner: "I'll send you a nude if you send me one."

A. Write your response.

_____

_____

_____

_____

_____

_____

_____

_____

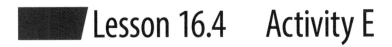 Lesson 16.4   Activity E

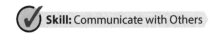

Assessing Your First-Aid Kit

Instructions: *Locate the first-aid kit or first-aid supplies in your home and assess which supplies you have and which ones are still needed. Ask a parent or guardian to help you, if needed. Indicate whether a supply is damaged or a medication is expired, if applicable. After assessing your first-aid kit and supplies, answer the reflection questions.*

First-Aid Kit

1. First-aid manual

   A. Got it? _____   C. Comments: _____

   B. Need it? _____   _____

2. Important phone numbers (doctor's office, etc.)

   A. Got it? _____   C. Comments: _____

   B. Need it? _____   _____

3. Gauze pads and assorted bandages

   A. Got it? _____   C. Comments: _____

   B. Need it? _____   _____

4. Medical tape

   A. Got it? _____   C. Comments: _____

   B. Need it? _____   _____

5. Cotton balls and cotton swabs

   A. Got it? _____   C. Comments: _____

   B. Need it? _____   _____

6. Scissors

   A. Got it? _____   C. Comments: _____

   B. Need it? _____   _____

7. Antibiotic ointment (cream)

   A. Got it? _____   C. Comments: _____

   B. Need it? _____   _____

8. Antiseptic wipes

   A. Got it? _____   C. Comments: _____

   B. Need it? _____   _____

9. Hand sanitizer

   A. Got it? _____   C. Comments: _____

   B. Need it? _____   _____

10. Disposable latex or synthetic gloves

   A. Got it? _____   C. Comments: _____

   B. Need it? _____   _____

11. Elastic wrap

   A. Got it? _____   C. Comments: _____

   B. Need it? _____   _____

12. Instant cold packs

   A. Got it? _____   C. Comments: _____

   B. Need it? _____   _____

13. Tweezers

   A. Got it? _____   C. Comments: _____

   B. Need it? _____   _____

14. Sterile eye drops or eyewash solution

   A. Got it? _____   C. Comments: _____

   B. Need it? _____   _____

15. Oral thermometer

   A. Got it? _____   C. Comments: _____

   B. Need it? _____   _____

16. Pain relievers (ibuprofen or acetaminophen)

   A. Got it? _____   C. Comments: _____

   B. Need it? _____   _____

17. Hydrocortisone cream

   A. Got it? _____   C. Comments: _____

   B. Need it? _____   _____

18. Antihistamine medications

   A. Got it? _____   C. Comments: _____

   B. Need it? _____   _____

Questions

1. What was the condition of your first-aid kit? Were the supplies neatly organized or scattered throughout the house?

   _____

   _____

2. Based on your current first-aid kit, do you feel prepared to respond to minor injuries or illnesses? Defend your answer. If not, what else is needed for you to successfully respond?

   _____

   _____

   _____

Chapter 16   Activity F

Practice Test

Completion

Instructions: *Write the term that completes the statement in the space provided.*

1. Practices that ensure health and safety during the performance of a task are _____.

_____

2. The _____ is a model that can help you remember the three elements needed to start a fire.

_____

3. A digital _____ includes all of the content people share, access, or have shared about them online.

_____

4. Drawing others into arguments and disrupting discussions online is called _____.

_____

5. Infection control practices called _____ were developed by the CDC to prevent the spread of disease during first aid.

_____

True/False

Instructions: *Indicate whether each statement below is true or false.*

6. _____ *True or false?* If you see a weapon such as a firearm, you should pick up the weapon and bring it to a trusted adult.

7. _____ *True or false?* The Occupational Safety and Health Act protects workers from dangers and hazards in the workplace and gives them rights.

8. _____ *True or false?* Because natural disasters are related to the weather, people cannot prepare for them.

9. _____ *True or false?* People have anonymity online, meaning law enforcement, officials, and employers cannot trace a person's online identity.

10. _____ *True or false?* Deep cuts, puncture wounds, or scratches can be treated at home without professional medical attention.

Multiple Choice

Instructions: *Select the letter that corresponds to the correct answer.*

11. _____ Which of the following is an effective strategy for safety on school buses?
    A. Always walk behind the school bus to get on.
    B. Wear your seat belt if available.
    C. If you drop something near a school bus, quickly pick it up.
    D. None of the above.

12. _____ Which of the following procedures can help you stay safe in the event of a fire?
    A. Crawl near to the floor to escape smoke and fumes.
    B. Identify one way to get out of each room.
    C. Make sure all bedrooms have no windows.
    D. Call 911 and then get out of the building.

13. _____ Which of the following do copyright laws protect?
    A. purchasing and downloading music
    B. watching a TV show online
    C. reposting content on social media
    D. All of the above.

14. _____ Which of the following methods makes a password strong?
    A. use of either uppercase or lowercase
    B. four to eight characters
    C. obvious personal information
    D. other keyboard characters (such as @ # $!)

15. _____ Burns are common injuries that can be caused by exposure to _____.
    A. fire or steam
    B. chemicals or electric current
    C. the sun
    D. All of the above.

Matching

Instructions: *Match each key term to its definition (16–21).*

16. _____ pretending to represent companies or government agencies and asking for personal information

17. _____ any object used to cause damage to an object or person

18. _____ severe allergic response in which fluid fills the lungs and air passages narrow

19. _____ right of a creator to exclusively own original material and use it in any way

20. _____ life-threatening condition in which the vital organs do not receive enough blood and oxygen

21. _____ writing mean and hateful comments with the intention of hurting others

A. anaphylaxis
B. copyright
C. flaming
D. phishing
E. shock
F. weapon

Analyzing Data

Instructions: *Use the data provided by the National Safety Council to answer the following questions.*

National Safety Council

Figure 1. Number of motor vehicle deaths in the US by year

22. Seat belts have been mandatory equipment in vehicles since 1968. What was the trend for motor vehicle deaths generally before 1968? after 1968?

_____

23. In 2018, for the first time in three years, fewer than 40,000 people died in motor vehicle crashes. What do you think is helping to curb motor vehicle crashes?

_____

Short Answer

Instructions: *Answer the following questions using what you have learned in this chapter.*

24. List three strategies to avoid using your phone while driving.

_____

_____

25. Explain when you can slow down or stop performing CPR.

_____

_____

Environmental Health

Lesson 17.1   Activity A

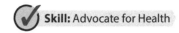 **Skill:** Advocate for Health

Advocating for the Environment

Instructions: *Reflect on and research ways that governments around the world can promote a healthier relationship between humans and the environment. Write a letter to US lawmakers to encourage legislation that promotes environmental action. Use the guide below to outline your message.*

1. Who is a US lawmaker you believe can make a difference in the legislation that might affect the environment? Explain.

   _____

   _____

   _____

2. How can you contact this person?

   _____

   _____

3. What benefits can positive environmentalism laws have on the general population?

   _____

   _____

   _____

   _____

4. What benefits can positive environmentalism laws have on the environment?

   _____

   _____

   _____

   _____

5. What strategies do you think can make a positive impact on the environment? List at least three.

   _____

   _____

   _____

   _____

   _____

Instructions: *Write your letter to this person using the benefits and strategies outlined above. Make sure to be clear, use appropriate language, and thank the person for their time. Send this letter to the person.*

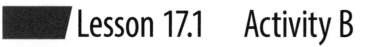 # Lesson 17.1   Activity B

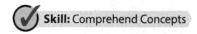

The Effects of Pollution

Instructions: *Examine the following scenarios about families who have encountered environmental hazards. Answer the questions following each scenario.*

Scenario 1

Last week, authorities temporarily shut off access to the water on the Jones family's whole block. They told Mrs. Jones that a farm in town had been using fertilizer to increase crop production and pesticides to deter bugs. These chemicals washed into a local stream during heavy rain. The local stream serves as a source of water in the Jones' neighborhood.

1. Which environmental hazard has the Jones family encountered?

_____

_____

2. How can this environmental hazard be prevented to reduce harm to people?

_____

_____

Scenario 2

Mr. Washington's son and daughter both work for him at his construction company. Much of this work involves spending time around loud construction vehicles and equipment, such as power tools. Recently, Mr. Washington's son complained about a ringing in his ears.

1. Which environmental hazard has the Washington family encountered?

_____

_____

2. How can this environmental hazard negatively affect a person's health?

_____

_____

Scenario 3

Mrs. Lee loves living in the city and has never considered moving. Recently, however, she married Mr. Lee and gained two new stepsons. When the Lees moved into her city apartment with her, the smog irritated them a lot. Mrs. Lee worries about the health effects of the smog.

1. Which environmental hazard has the Lee family encountered?

_____

_____

2. How could the smog affect the Lee family?

_____

_____

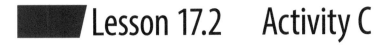 Lesson 17.2 Activity C 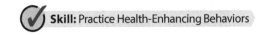 **Skill:** Practice Health-Enhancing Behaviors

Safe Chemical Use

Instructions: *Read the following scenarios about people who have been exposed to hazardous chemicals. Rewrite the scenarios to show how each person can eliminate this risk.*

1. Eli knows he is supposed to include eight ounces of cooked seafood in his diet each week. He chooses fish that contain mercury to eat.

   A. Rewrite the scenario showing how Eli can eliminate the risk of chemicals.

   _____

   _____

   _____

   _____

2. Aisha drinks her coffee in the morning out of a container made with BPA.

   A. Rewrite the scenario showing how Aisha can eliminate the risk of chemicals.

   _____

   _____

   _____

   _____

3. To effectively sanitize the bathroom, Mr. Garcia uses a solution of bleach and ammonia.

   A. Rewrite the scenario showing how Mr. Garcia can eliminate the risk of chemicals.

   _____

   _____

   _____

   _____

4. Pete's family tested the paint in their new house for lead. The lead levels are unsafe, so they start the process of removing the paint themselves.

   A. Rewrite the scenario showing how Pete's family can eliminate the risk of chemicals.

   _____

   _____

   _____

   _____

5. Mrs. Miller sprays her grass with herbicides to kill and prevent weeds. Shortly after, her young son plays barefoot in the grass.

   A. Rewrite the scenario showing how Mrs. Miller can eliminate the risk of chemicals.

   _____

   _____

   _____

   _____

6. On Friday night, Lucas invites his friends over for a bonfire. For firewood, Lucas cuts up an old dresser made out of pressure-treated wood.

   A. Rewrite the scenario showing how Lucas can eliminate the risk of chemicals.

   _____

   _____

   _____

   _____

7. Mrs. Johnson sprays her vegetable garden with a pesticide to deter bugs. Then, she picks a tomato to eat while pulling weeds.

   A. Rewrite the scenario showing how Mrs. Johnson can eliminate the risk of chemicals.

   _____

   _____

   _____

   _____

8. Kara lives near an open field where her fire department practices controlling forest fires. She is concerned about the PFAS levels in her water.

   A. Rewrite the scenario showing how Kara can eliminate the risk of chemicals.

   _____

   _____

   _____

   _____

Name _____ Date _____ Period _____

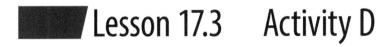 Lesson 17.3   Activity D

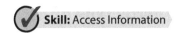

Renewable Energy

Instructions: *Renewable energy comes from sources such as wind, water, and sunlight, which do not run out. It also does not cause pollution. Using reliable resources, conduct research about two types of renewable energy. Use the questions to focus your research.*

Energy Type #1

1. Which type of renewable energy did you choose?

   _____

2. How does this type of renewable energy work?

   _____

   _____

3. What are some recent developments in this renewable energy?

   _____

   _____

   _____

   _____

   _____

   _____

4. How much does this type of energy cost?

   _____

5. What are the limitations of this type of energy?

   _____

   _____

   _____

   _____

6. What are the benefits of using this type of energy?

   _____

   _____

   _____

   _____

7. Provide a citation for one of the reliable resources you used for your research. Include the article title, author, information sponsor, and publication date.

   _____

   _____

   _____

Energy Type #2

1. Which type of renewable energy did you choose?

_____

2. How does this type of renewable energy work?

_____

_____

3. What are some recent developments in this renewable energy?

_____

_____

_____

_____

_____

_____

4. How much does this type of energy cost?

_____

5. What are the limitations of this type of energy?

_____

_____

_____

_____

6. What are the benefits of using this type of energy?

_____

_____

_____

_____

7. Provide a citation for one of the reliable resources you used for your research. Include the article title, author, information sponsor, and publication date.

_____

_____

_____

_____

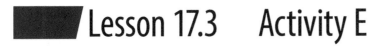 Lesson 17.3   Activity E

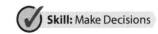 **Skill:** Make Decisions

The Environmental Protection Hierarchy

Instructions: *Review the environmental protection hierarchy shown in the text. Then, examine the following scenarios and decide on a greener option that would help protect the environment. Also state which strategy of the hierarchy you used: source reduction, reuse, recycling, or treatment and disposal.*

1. The remote for Jayzon's TV needs new batteries. At the store, he buys a pack of AAA batteries.

   A. List a greener option: _____

   _____

   B. Identify the environmental protection hierarchy strategy: _____

   _____

2. Daniela is at the grocery store and is offered paper or plastic bags for her groceries. She accepts plastic.

   A. List a greener option: _____

   _____

   B. Identify the environmental protection hierarchy strategy: _____

   _____

3. Madeline goes to the grocery store and buys fruits and vegetables that have been imported from all over the world.

   A. List a greener option: _____

   _____

   B. Identify the environmental protection hierarchy strategy: _____

   _____

4. Brian throws an aerosol can of household cleaner in the trash because it expired.

   A. List a greener option: _____

   _____

   B. Identify the environmental protection hierarchy strategy: _____

   _____

5. Every day, Braden throws his empty sparkling water can away in the trash.

   A. List a greener option: _____

   _____

   B. Identify the environmental protection hierarchy strategy: _____

   _____

6. While repairing his car, Neil throws away the old tires and car battery.

   A. List a greener option: _____

   _____

   B. Identify the environmental protection hierarchy strategy: _____

   _____

7. Based on his wife's request, Marcel buys a car that uses 87 octane gas, which is the cheapest grade of gasoline.

   A. List a greener option: _____

   _____

   B. Identify the environmental protection hierarchy strategy: _____

   _____

8. Janessa just bought a new laptop. Her old computer is small enough to dispose of in the garbage can.

   A. List a greener option: _____

   _____

   B. Identify the environmental protection hierarchy strategy: _____

   _____

9. Sometimes, Aiden and his family make too much food for dinner and have to throw away the extras.

   A. List a greener option: _____

   _____

   B. Identify the environmental protection hierarchy strategy: _____

   _____

10. Lexi brings her lunch to school every day using disposable plastic and brown paper bags.

    A. List a greener option: _____

    _____

    B. Identify the environmental protection hierarchy strategy: _____

    _____

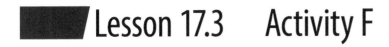 Lesson 17.3   Activity F

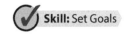 **Skill:** Set Goals

Greener Living

Instructions: *Consider what you can do in your daily life to go green. Then, list five realistic strategies you can do each day that will help you achieve your goal of protecting the environment. Record your progress for one week. Then, answer the reflection questions.*

Strategies

1. Strategy: _____
   _____
   _____

   A. _____   Monday
   B. _____   Tuesday
   C. _____   Wednesday
   D. _____   Thursday
   E. _____   Friday
   F. _____   Saturday
   G. _____   Sunday

2. Strategy: _____
   _____
   _____

   A. _____   Monday
   B. _____   Tuesday
   C. _____   Wednesday
   D. _____   Thursday
   E. _____   Friday
   F. _____   Saturday
   G. _____   Sunday

3. Strategy: _____
   _____
   _____

   A. _____   Monday
   B. _____   Tuesday
   C. _____   Wednesday
   D. _____   Thursday
   E. _____   Friday
   F. _____   Saturday
   G. _____   Sunday

4. Strategy: _____

_____

_____

    A. _____ Monday

    B. _____ Tuesday

    C. _____ Wednesday

    D. _____ Thursday

    E. _____ Friday

    F. _____ Saturday

    G. _____ Sunday

5. Strategy: _____

_____

_____

    A. _____ Monday

    B. _____ Tuesday

    C. _____ Wednesday

    D. _____ Thursday

    E. _____ Friday

    F. _____ Saturday

    G. _____ Sunday

Questions

1. After one week of greener living, which strategy were you most successful in implementing? least successful?

_____

_____

_____

2. What factors contributed to how well you met your goal each day?

_____

_____

_____

3. How will achieving your goal each day positively affect the environment?

_____

_____

_____

4. What adjustment or changes would you make to your strategies to stay motivated and continue to strive to make a difference?

_____

_____

_____

▰ Chapter 17   Activity G

Practice Test

Completion

Instructions: *Write the term that completes the statement in the space provided.*

1. Biotic parts of _____ include the living parts while the abiotic parts include nonliving aspects like water, air, sunlight, and temperature.

   _____

2. _____ occurs if forests are removed faster than they regrow.

   _____

3. An element normally found in soils and rocks, _____ is poisonous and carcinogenic at high levels.

   _____

4. _____ energy is created using natural materials, such as when garbage rots in a landfill.

   _____

5. A great way to reduce waste is to _____ by throwing food scraps into a bin or pile separate from the trash to break down over time.

   _____

True/False

Instructions: *Indicate whether each statement below is true or false.*

6. _____ *True or false?* The natural environment, not your built environment, affects your environmental health.

7. _____ *True or false?* As a population grows, it consumes more resources and produces more waste.

8. _____ *True or false?* Bisphenol A is a chemical used to make plastic and may be harmful to humans.

9. _____ *True or false?* The Environmental Protection Agency (EPA) finds all approaches to protecting the environment equally preferred.

10. _____ *True or false?* Bottles, cans, newspapers, TVs, computers, and appliances can all be recycled in the same way.

Multiple Choice

Instructions: *Select the letter that corresponds to the correct answer.*

11. _____ Which of the following is *not* an example of a natural resource?
    A. sunlight   C. electricity
    B. fossil fuels   D. minerals

12. _____ Which of the following natural events and sources causes air pollution?
    A. litter   C. pesticides and herbicides
    B. noise from airplanes   D. fuel emissions

13. _____ Which of the following EPA laws provides rules and regulations for managing hazardous wastes?
    A. Brownfield Site Act   C. Resource Conservation and Recovery Act
    B. Safe Drinking Water Act   D. Clean Air Act

14. _____ Which of the following benefits is true of planting a tree?
    A. traps dust and pollen from the air   C. reduces water runoff from storms
    B. reduces heat buildup during the day   D. All of the above.

Matching

Instructions: *Match each key term to its definition (15–20).*

15. _____ widespread hunger and starvation caused by lack of food

16. _____ chemicals that evaporate in the air and can cause several health issues

17. _____ natural mineral in soils; can cause cancer when inhaled

18. _____ silver metal that is liquid at room temperature

19. _____ extended period with no rainfall

20. _____ chemicals used to destroy insects or other organisms that harm plants or animals

A. asbestos

B. drought

C. famine

D. mercury

E. pesticides

F. volatile organic compounds (VOCs)

Analyzing Data

Instructions: *Read the following data from the US Energy Information Administration. Use the information provided to answer the following questions.*

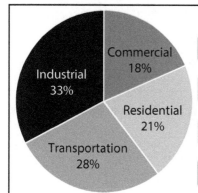

Share of Total US Energy Consumption by Sector

The industrial sector includes facilities and equipment used for manufacturing, agriculture, mining, and construction.

The transportation sector includes vehicles that transport people or goods, such as cars, trucks, buses, trains, aircraft, boats, barges, and ships.

The residential sector includes homes and apartments and their individual uses of heating, cooling, appliances, and electronics.

The commercial sector includes offices, malls, stores, schools, hospitals, hotels, warehouses, and restaurants.

US Energy Information Administration

Figure 1. Total US energy consumption

21. Which sector uses the most energy in the US? the least?

_____

22. If a large portion of energy use in the residential sector goes toward heating and cooling homes, what can people do to reduce energy consumption?

_____

_____

Short Answer

Instructions: *Answer the following questions using what you have learned in this chapter.*

23. What do greenhouse gases do for Earth's atmosphere? What is currently happening with Earth's greenhouse gases?

_____

_____

24. Give four examples of green products you can buy and use that have a less harmful impact on the environment than their traditional counterparts.

_____

_____

_____

CHAPTER 18 Communicable Diseases

Lesson 18.1   Activity A

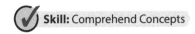

Skill: Comprehend Concepts

The Life of a Pathogen

Instructions: *Read the following descriptions to determine which pathogen is present. Then, answer the questions that follow.*

Descriptions

1. I am a single-celled organism that lives in nearly every possible place.

   A. Identify the type of pathogen: _____

2. I live inside a cell and use that cell's resources and energy to grow and reproduce.

   A. Identify the type of pathogen: _____

3. I make up 90 percent of your cells. I am everywhere, but most of the time I am helpful.

   A. Identify the type of pathogen: _____

4. I am an organism that contains cells specialized for feeding, anchoring to surfaces, and producing spores for reproduction.

   A. Identify the type of pathogen: _____

5. As an egg, I was living in contaminated water. When you drank that water, I started to grow in your intestine.

   A. Identify the type of pathogen: _____

6. Once inside the body, I will invade your cells and direct them to create more of me.

   A. Identify the type of pathogen: _____

7. I caused your food poisoning. I was in the undercooked burger you ate for lunch.

   A. Identify the type of pathogen: _____

8. I caused your athlete's foot. I live on the moist surfaces in your pool's shower, locker room, and pool deck.

   A. Identify the type of pathogen: _____

9. I cause some of the world's most feared diseases such as malaria and dysentery.

   A. Identify the type of pathogen: _____

Questions

1. Which life-saving drug that controls bacterial infections is made from a fungus? _____

2. Which type of pathogen is *Staphylococcus aureus*? What health condition is caused by this pathogen?

   _____

3. What type of pathogen is hookworm? What health consequences can occur with the growth of a hookworm in the body?

   _____

4. Which type of pathogen causes HIV/AIDS, COVID-19, measles, and chicken pox? _____

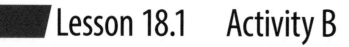 Lesson 18.1   Activity B   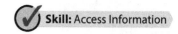 **Skill:** Access Information

Finding Reliable Health Information

Instructions: *Conduct research using reliable resources to answer the following questions about your choice of pathogen: bacteria, viruses, fungi, or parasites. Provide citations for your sources and defend their reliability.*

1. What type of pathogen will you research?

   _____

2. Provide a description of this type of pathogen and how it interacts with the body.

   _____

   _____

3. List three strains of this type of pathogen.

   _____

   _____

   _____

4. How is this type of pathogen typically transmitted? Explain.

   _____

   _____

   _____

   _____

5. List citations for your sources of information.

   A. Source #1

      Name of organization: _____

      Title of article or page: _____

      Author name: _____

   B. Source #2

      Name of organization: _____

      Title of article or page: _____

      Author name: _____

6. Reflect on your sources. Which source was more reliable? How do you know?

   _____

   _____

   _____

   _____

   _____

   _____

   _____

   _____

Name _____ Date _____ Period _____

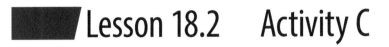 Lesson 18.2   Activity C

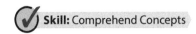

Signs and Symptoms

Instructions: *For each scenario presented, differentiate between the signs and symptoms for each patient. If a patient does not exhibit either signs or symptoms, write "N/A." Identify the communicable disease in each scenario and list which type of pathogen is responsible for this condition.*

1. Kaden has a headache, fever (temperature of 101° F), and sore throat.

   A. What are the signs? _____

   _____

   B. What are the symptoms? _____

   _____

   C. Identify the disease: _____

   D. Identify the pathogen responsible: _____

2. LaShara has a runny nose, and she has been sneezing and coughing.

   A. What are the signs? _____

   _____

   B. What are the symptoms? _____

   _____

   C. Identify the disease: _____

   D. Identify the pathogen responsible: _____

3. Following a swim meet, Tyler's feet start to itch and burn. He develops a rash between his toes.

   A. What are the signs? _____

   _____

   B. What are the symptoms? _____

   _____

   C. Identify the disease: _____

   D. Identify the pathogen responsible: _____

4. Eve's stomach hurts and her urine is dark. Her skin is also yellow and itchy. Her liver is failing.

   A. What are the signs? _____

   _____

   B. What are the symptoms? _____

   _____

   C. Identify the disease: _____

   D. Identify the pathogen responsible: _____

5. Harrison woke up with a fever and a dry cough. He noticed the coffee he drank this morning did not smell right and barely had any taste.

    A. What are the signs? _____

    _____

    B. What are the symptoms? _____

    _____

    C. Identify the disease: _____

    D. Identify the pathogen responsible: _____

6. Gabriela's throat hurts a lot. She has a fever, and her tonsils are swollen.

    A. What are the signs? _____

    _____

    B. What are the symptoms? _____

    _____

    C. Identify the disease: _____

    D. Identify the pathogen responsible: _____

7. Alejandro feels tired all the time. He has a fever and sore throat, and his doctor says his spleen is swollen.

    A. What are the signs? _____

    _____

    B. What are the symptoms? _____

    _____

    C. Identify the disease: _____

    D. Identify the pathogen responsible: _____

8. When Jackie first woke up, she had a hard time opening her eye. Her eye is red, itchy, and watery.

    A. What are the signs? _____

    _____

    B. What are the symptoms? _____

    _____

    C. Identify the disease: _____

    D. Identify the pathogen responsible: _____

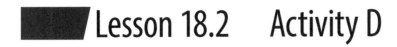 Lesson 18.2   Activity D

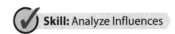 **Skill:** Analyze Influences

Emerging Infectious Diseases

Instructions: *In your own words, define epidemic, pandemic, and endemic. Then, read each scenario about emerging infectious diseases and determine what factor may influence this emergence.*

1. Define *epidemic*.

_____

_____

_____

2. Define *pandemic*.

_____

_____

_____

3. Define *endemic*.

_____

_____

_____

Scenarios

1. A mosquito-borne disease naturally occurs at low levels in a particular area. This area, experiencing more floods this season, is seeing an increase in this disease.

   A. Identify the influencing factor: _____

2. Over the last few decades, a certain disease has been regularly and successfully treated with antibiotics. This disease now does not respond to these medications.

   A. Identify the influencing factor: _____

3. A fungus that is common among patients in hospitals is typically treated with a drug. Recently, the fungus has not gone away when treated with this drug.

   A. Identify the influencing factor: _____

4. A new species of tick has been discovered in a certain area. With it, a new disease transmitted by tick bites has been introduced to the area as well.

   A. Identify the influencing factor: _____

5. When a vaccine for a disease was discovered, cases of this disease nearly disappeared. Certain communities have stopped getting this vaccine, and the disease has begun to re-emerge.

   A. Identify the influencing factor: _____

Lesson 18.3   Activity E

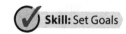

Setting Disease-Prevention Goals

Instructions: *Develop a SMART goal to improve your health practices that prevent communicable diseases. This SMART goal should help you maintain or improve your personal health in this area. Use the following statements/questions to outline your SMART goal.*

Outline Your SMART Goal

1. Assess your personal health practices relating to communicable disease prevention.

   _____

   _____

2. Identify a basic goal for maintaining or improving your health in this area.

   _____

3. State what you would like to achieve. Be **specific**.

   _____

   _____

4. How will you **measure** whether or not you have achieved this goal?

   _____

5. Set short-term goals to help make your large goal more **achievable**.

   _____

   _____

6. How is this goal **relevant** to your current identity and values?

   _____

7. Set a **time line** for completing your goal. Set dates for your short-term goals and your larger goal.

   _____

   _____

8. How will you act on this goal? Whom will you ask for support?

   _____

9. How will you monitor your progress?

   _____

10. What obstacles might keep you from reaching your goal? How can you overcome these obstacles?

    _____

    _____

Write Your SMART Goal

1. Summarize the information above as your comprehensive SMART goal.

   _____

Name _____ Date _____ Period _____

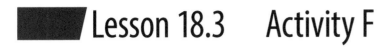 Lesson 18.3　　Activity F

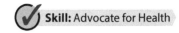 Skill: Advocate for Health

Epidemics and Public Health

Instructions: *Read the following story about the 1918 influenza pandemic.*

An estimated one third of the world's population became infected with an influenza virus during 1918 and 1919. There was no vaccine to protect against influenza at the time. In addition, antibiotics did not exist to treat secondary bacterial infections from influenza. Control efforts included isolation, quarantine, personal hygiene, and use of disinfectants.

Instructions: *Conduct research using reliable resources about an epidemic or pandemic from the last two years. Answer the following questions to find out how individuals and a community can promote health in the face of an infectious disease.*

1. Name the epidemic and explain the signs and symptoms of this disease.

_____

_____

_____

_____

_____

_____

_____

2. What type of pathogen causes this disease? How is this disease transmitted?

_____

_____

_____

_____

3. How can medical professionals treat this disease? Is a vaccine available?

_____

_____

_____

_____

_____

4. What can individuals in a community do to prevent the spread of this disease? Name at least four behaviors.

_____

_____

_____

_____

_____

_____

_____

5. What did organizations or governments do to facilitate prevention and treatment methods? What more could they have done?

_____

_____

_____

_____

_____

_____

_____

_____

_____

_____

Instructions: *Create a campaign to present information about this infectious disease to students and adults at your school. This campaign can use whatever medium you choose, such as social media posts, posters, emails, presentations, or flyers.*

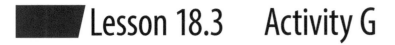 Lesson 18.3   Activity G   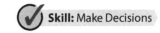 Skill: Make Decisions

Rewrite the Story

Instructions: *Read the scenarios about Kailani, Thomas, Trinity, and José. As you are reading, identify unhealthy behaviors that could increase the risk of communicable diseases. Then, rewrite their stories by changing their decisions and adding strategies to prevent these diseases.*

Scenario 1

> Kailani has perfect attendance at school, so when she gets the flu, she goes to school as soon as her fever breaks. She is still coughing and sneezing a lot, but she tries to always cough or sneeze into her hands. If she uses a tissue, she stores it in her pocket until she can get home to dispose of it. She avoids washing her hands because she does not want to spread her germs on the faucet in the bathroom.

1. What unhealthy behaviors put Kailani at risk of spreading a communicable disease to others at school?

   _____

   _____

   _____

2. Rewrite Kailani's story to change these unhealthy behaviors. Include three or more steps Kailani can take to prevent others from getting a communicable disease.

   _____

   _____

   _____

   _____

   _____

   _____

Scenario 2

> Thomas knows he needs to take better care of himself. He eats a lot of junk food and drinks alcohol with his friends. He spends multiple hours after school playing video games, and then stays up late cramming for upcoming quizzes. This means he rarely gets more than five or six hours of sleep at night. Thomas has not been to the doctor in a few years, but he knows his doctor would probably tell him he needs to get more physical activity.

1. What unhealthy behaviors put Thomas at risk of developing a communicable disease?

   _____

   _____

   _____

2. Rewrite Thomas' story to change these unhealthy behaviors. Include four or more steps Thomas can take to reduce his risk of developing communicable diseases.

   _____

   _____

   _____

   _____

Scenario 3

> Trinity has a fear of needles. She tries to stay healthy as much as she can so she can avoid going to the doctor. Trinity does not get her flu shot each year because of her fear of needles. She knows she got other vaccines that she needed for school, but has not gotten any follow-up booster shots since then.

1. What unhealthy behaviors put Trinity at risk of developing a communicable disease?

   _____

   _____

   _____

2. Rewrite Trinity's story to change these unhealthy behaviors. Include steps Trinity can take to reduce her risk of developing communicable diseases.

   _____

   _____

   _____

   _____

   _____

   _____

Scenario 4

> José has a common cold, but his doctor told him that he could continue going to school. His doctor warned José to cover his mouth and nose when he sneezes and coughs, and to wash his hands more frequently. José always washes his hands for 10 seconds or so after he uses the bathroom, and he figures that is often enough. He really only rubs his palms and fronts of his fingers, since that is what he would cough or sneeze on. Once, the bathroom was out of soap, so José just rinsed his hands in warm water.

1. What unhealthy behaviors put José at risk of developing a communicable disease?

   _____

   _____

   _____

2. Rewrite José's story to change these unhealthy behaviors. Include steps José can take to reduce his risk of developing communicable diseases.

   _____

   _____

   _____

   _____

   _____

   _____

Chapter 18   Activity H

Practice Test

Completion

Instructions: *Write the term that completes the statement in the space provided.*

1. Germ theory states that disease-causing microorganisms, called _____, cause specific diseases.

   _____

2. _____ are evidence of disease that can be outwardly observed or measured.

   _____

3. _____ are evidence of disease sensed by the person with the disease.

   _____

4. The only proven method of successfully eliminating a communicable disease is _____.

   _____

5. For infections such as hepatitis and severe influenza, _____ medications can reduce the severity of the infection and risk of transmission.

   _____

True/False

Instructions: *Indicate whether each statement below is true or false.*

6. _____ *True or false?* Bacteria, viruses, fungi, and phagocytes are examples of pathogens.

7. _____ *True or false?* Most bacteria are *not* harmful to the body.

8. _____ *True or false?* During the *clinical stage*, a pathogen produces toxins and the immune response reaches its height, causing familiar signs of illness.

9. _____ *True or false?* In the *convalescent stage*, signs and symptoms of an illness gradually worsen.

Multiple Choice

Instructions: *Select the letter that corresponds to the correct answer.*

10. _____ Which of the following is true about viruses?
    - A. Viruses do not grow or reproduce independently.
    - B. Viruses have no metabolism.
    - C. Viruses do not use energy in the way that other cells do.
    - D. All of the above.

11. _____ When a _____ infection develops, it is called mycosis, and it usually affects damaged tissues or people weakened by other infections.
    - A. bacterial
    - B. viral
    - C. fungal
    - D. parasitical

12. _____ Which of the following is an example of a parasite?
    - A. *Ascaris lumbricoides*
    - B. *Staphylococcus aureus*
    - C. *Penicillium notatum*
    - D. *Pneumocystis jirovecii*

13. _____ Parasitic worms are _____ organisms with specialized tissues and organs.
    - A. single-celled
    - B. quadricellular
    - C. dual-celled
    - D. multicellular

Matching

Instructions: *Match each key term to its definition (14–21).*

14. _____ dangerous disease caused by a strain of the *S. aureus* bacterium that is resistant to the antibiotic methicillin

15. _____ medications that target and kill disease-causing bacteria

16. _____ disease that spreads to much of the world

17. _____ disease that occurs in unexpectedly large numbers over a particular area

18. _____ behaviors that prevent the spread of disease through droplets

19. _____ substance containing a dead pathogen or nontoxic part of a pathogen; introduced into the body to provoke an immune response

20. _____ disease that naturally occurs in low levels in a particular area

21. _____ practice of using soap and water to clean the hands

A. antibiotics

B. endemic

C. epidemic

D. hand washing

E. MRSA

F. pandemic

G. respiratory etiquette

H. vaccine

Analyzing Data

Instructions: *Use the data provided by the Centers for Disease Control and Prevention about the 2018–2019 influenza season to answer the questions that follow.*

Age Group	Symptomatic Illnesses	Medical Visits	Hospitalizations	Deaths
0–4 years	10.2%	14.7%	5.2%	0.8%
5–17 years	21.6%	24.1%	4.3%	0.6%
18–49 years	33.5%	26.7%	13.6%	7.2%
50–64 years	26.0%	24.0%	20.0%	16.6%
65+ years	8.7%	10.4%	57.0%	74.8%

Centers for Disease Control and Prevention

Figure 1. Data from the 2018–2019 influenza season

22. Which age group has the highest rate of illnesses symptomatic with influenza? _____

23. Which age group has the highest rates of hospitalizations from influenza?_____

Short Answer

Instructions: *Answer the following questions using what you have learned in this chapter.*

24. Summarize the difference between the *direct transmission* and *indirect transmission* of a communicable disease. Give two examples of each transmission method.

_____

_____

25. List four behaviors that can help promote resistance of infection by supporting your immune system.

_____

_____

_____

26. Briefly define the term *vaccine* and give at least three examples of a vaccine.

_____

_____

_____

CHAPTER 19 / Sexually Transmitted Infections and HIV/AIDS

Lesson 19.1   Activity A

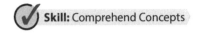

STI Transmission

Instructions: *In each of the following scenarios, explain why an STI could or could not have been transmitted.*

1. The night after Ciara and Jim kiss for the first time, Ciara texts her friend to tell her the news. Ciara's friend wants to be excited for her, but she also has some bad news. She knows that Jim has *herpes*, which can sometimes manifest as sores on the mouth.

   A. Could an STI have been transmitted? Why or why not?

   _____

   _____

   _____

   _____

2. Travis and Natalia have discussed sex and decide that they are both ready. During their discussions, Travis says he has been sexually active in the past and recently tested positive for *HPV*. When they have sex, Travis and Natalia use a latex condom and dental dam.

   A. Could an STI have been transmitted? Why or why not?

   _____

   _____

   _____

   _____

3. Molly and Jen are hanging out at their friend Dexter's house. While there, Molly uses the bathroom. After they leave Dexter's house, Jen tells Molly that Dexter has *gonorrhea*. Molly is worried because she used the same toilet seat that Dexter has used in the past.

   A. Could an STI have been transmitted? Why or why not?

   _____

   _____

   _____

   _____

4. Lindsay and Isaac have decided not to have sex yet because they do not feel ready to handle the risk of a pregnancy. They still do engage in other sexual activities, however.

   A. Could an STI have been transmitted? Why or why not?

   _____

   _____

   _____

   _____

Name _____ Date _____ Period _____

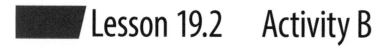 Lesson 19.2   Activity B

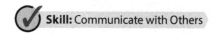

Abstinence

Instructions: *Read the following scenarios in which a person's choice to practice abstinence is challenged. In each situation, provide an example of a strong response that would convey a commitment to abstinence and the person's right to be respected.*

Scenario 1

Shondra and her boyfriend, Alex, have been dating for two years. When the relationship first began, Shondra was clear about her choice to practice abstinence. Alex seemed to agree with her at first, but then he began pressuring her to engage in sexual activity. He told Shondra that she should be ready by now since they had been dating for years.

1. How should Shondra respond?

_____

_____

Scenario 2

Eric and Marina have been dating all throughout high school. Although Eric knows that his relationship with Marina is solid and that they may get married one day, he has chosen to remain abstinent until then. Marina and Eric have discussed this before, and Marina has always seemed to agree with Eric. Graduation is approaching, however, and Marina mentions wanting to have sex on prom night to Eric.

1. What should Eric say?

_____

_____

Scenario 3

Bonnie and Colton have only been on four dates. Bonnie is committed to abstinence, but she has not yet talked about it with Colton. One evening, Colton mentions that her parents are away for the weekend. She invites Bonnie to stay the night at her house and implies that they could engage in sexual activity. Bonnie wants to hang out with Colton, but she does not want to put herself in a risky situation.

1. What should Bonnie say?

_____

_____

Scenario 4

Kali and Toby have been dating for a few years. One day, Kali's friends start discussing how they have already had sex with their boyfriends. Kali's friends ask why Kali and Toby have not had sex yet. Kali and Toby talked about this and have both decided to remain abstinent.

1. How could Kali explain this to her friends?

_____

_____

Name _____ Date _____ Period _____

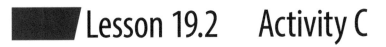 Lesson 19.2   Activity C

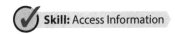

Health Information

Instructions: *Find a website or article that provides information about STIs, treatments, and prevention. Answer the following questions to evaluate if this resource is reliable, unbiased, and accurate.*

1. Provide a citation for the website or article you found. Include the website or article name, author, and sponsor.

    _____

    _____

    _____

2. Use the following checklist to evaluate the validity and reliability of your resource.

    A. _____ Information is current up to one year.

    B. _____ Information is supported by other reliable resources.

    C. _____ Information is based on scientific research.

    D. _____ There is adequate information about the topic.

    E. _____ Facts are cited or referenced.

    F. _____ Information is reasonable (not too good to be true).

    G. _____ Information is applicable to my life stage and situation.

    H. _____ Purpose of resource is stated.

    I. _____ Resource is not making money from the information (not an advertisement).

    J. _____ Author's name is listed.

    K. _____ Author's background is trustworthy and dependable.

    L. _____ Author presents unbiased information.

    M. _____ Resource is sponsored by a credible institution or organization.

    N. _____ Website address of resource ends in .gov, .edu, or .org.

3. After your evaluation, do you think your article is a reliable source of information? Explain.

    _____

    _____

    _____

    _____

    _____

    _____

    _____

4. Would you recommend other teens use this website? Why or why not?

    _____

    _____

    _____

    _____

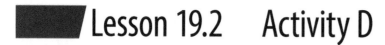 Lesson 19.2   Activity D

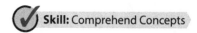 **Skill: Comprehend Concepts**

STI Test Results

Instructions: *Imagine that you are a doctor who is diagnosing a patient with an STI. Read each of the following descriptions of a patient's symptoms. Then, diagnose each person with an STI and explain what type of treatment is best suited for that specific STI.*

Patient 1

Bianca has a copper-colored rash on the palms of her hands and the soles of her feet. When asked, she reveals that she noticed a painless sore on her tongue three weeks ago. In addition to her rash, Bianca feels fatigued and has a mild fever. After an examination, you note that Bianca's lymph nodes are swollen.

1. Which STI does Bianca have? _____

2. What treatments are available?

_____

Patient 2

Gabby has noticed warts on her genitals and she tells you that she has been having unprotected sex with her dating partner. She is worried that she has contracted an STI like herpes. You are concerned about the genital warts, so you perform a Pap smear.

1. Which STI does Gabby have? _____

2. What treatments are available?

_____

Patient 3

A few weeks ago, Greg developed blisters on his genitals. He thought about seeing a doctor, but the blisters burst and healed. Greg now has these blisters again, but milder this time. He also has a low-grade fever.

1. Which STI does Greg have? _____

2. What treatments are available?

_____

Patient 4

Cathy has started experiencing nausea, abdominal pain, fever, and abnormal bleeding during her menstrual period. She also feels a burning sensation when she pees. Cathy thinks she may have contracted an STI when she had unprotected sex last summer. Until now, she has not experienced any symptoms.

1. Which STI does Cathy have? _____

2. What treatments are available?

_____

Name _____ Date _____ Period _____

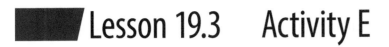
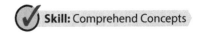
HIV Transmission

Instructions: *Read the following scenarios and determine whether the person should be worried about HIV transmission. Explain your answer.*

1. Heather's uncle has AIDS. After visiting, Heather's uncle kisses her on the cheek and gives her a hug goodbye.
   A. Can HIV have been transmitted? Explain.

   _____

   _____

2. Sanjay and Aaliyah are in a sexually active relationship. Both have had previous sexual partners and neither has been tested for HIV.
   A. Can HIV have been transmitted? Explain.

   _____

   _____

3. After her daughter was born, Diane contracted HIV. Diane thinks that breastfeeding is important, so she continues to breastfeed after her diagnosis.
   A. Can HIV have been transmitted? Explain.

   _____

   _____

4. Lara knows that Dominic has HIV. After going on a run together, Dominic and Lara share a water bottle to rehydrate.
   A. Can HIV have been transmitted? Explain.

   _____

   _____

5. Pedro has AIDS. Jill and Pedro have sexual intercourse and do not use a condom or other protective method.
   A. Can HIV have been transmitted? Explain.

   _____

   _____

6. Jeong works in a hospital emergency room. One day, a patient's blood gets onto a cut on Jeong's arm. He later finds out that patient has HIV.
   A. Can HIV have been transmitted? Explain.

   _____

   _____

7. Gavin knows that Harry has AIDS. One day, Gavin uses gym equipment that Harry just used, and he notices Harry's sweat on it.
   A. Can HIV have been transmitted? Explain.

   _____

   _____

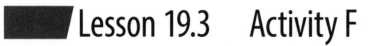 Lesson 19.3　Activity F

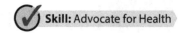

PEP and PrEP

Instructions: *In small groups, create an advertisement to inform people about the medications PEP and PrEP. Follow the instructions below to get started. Then, create your advertisement, using the medium of your choice, and share it with the class.*

Choose a target group.

1. Advertisements are crafted to appeal to a particular audience. Which group(s) of people will your PEP and PrEP advertisement target? Some target audiences might be teens, adults, women or men, people of a particular economic or ethnic group, or people who are or are not sexually active. Describe your target audience.

_____

_____

_____

_____

_____

_____

Choose a focus.

1. Choose a message you want to communicate. There is too much information about PEP and PrEP to include in a short advertisement. You need to narrow your focus. For example, you might focus on the use of PEP and PrEP among healthcare professionals or the fact that PEP and PrEP can protect a person from contracting HIV. Consider what kind of message will appeal to the group you have chosen. Summarize the message of your ad.

_____

_____

_____

_____

_____

_____

Choose a medium for your message.

1. Choose a medium for your advertisement. Your group might create a flyer, poster, video, podcast, or website. When choosing your medium, consider which medium will best reach your target audience. Describe which medium your group chose and why you chose it.

_____

_____

_____

_____

_____

_____

Name _____ Date _____ Period _____

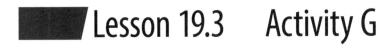 Lesson 19.3   Activity G   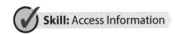 Skill: Access Information

Health Careers

Instructions: *When choosing a healthcare career, be mindful of your personal interests, strengths, and weaknesses. These will help you decide which career would best suit you. Study the information in the chart and answer the questions that follow. Do additional research as needed to complete the activity.*

Career	Interest/Quality	Duties	Education and Training	Resource
Medical laboratory technologist	Enjoys working with people in a fast-paced environment An interest in science	Collects blood and tissue samples from patients, performs tests, and analyzes results in a timely manner	Bachelor's degree, certification, or licensure	American Society for Clinical Laboratory Science
Community health worker	Enjoys working with the public Good communication skills	Conducts community outreach programs Educates the public about health concerns	Associate's degree and/or certification	American Public Health Association
Health information technician	Enjoys working with data or paperwork Enjoys working independently Good communication skills	Organizes, maintains, and records patient health data Works with patient data rather than directly with patients Reports cases of STIs per hospital guidelines	Associate's degree and/or certification	American Health Information Management Association
Microbiologist	Enjoys working with data or paperwork Enjoys working independently An interest in science Ability to meet deadlines	Studies microorganisms, such as those that cause STIs, and records data Spends time analyzing data in the lab and presents data and findings in a timely manner	Bachelor's degree and/or master's degree or PhD	American Society for Microbiology

Figure 1. Information about sexual health careers

1. Which of these careers most interests you? Explain why you think this career suits your interests and personal qualities.

_____

_____

_____

_____

_____

_____

_____

_____

_____

_____

_____

2. Research this career further. Visit the resource listed in the chart for that career and compose a "day in the life" for someone with that career. Does this type of workday sound interesting to you?

_____

_____

_____

_____

_____

3. According to the chart, what level of education is necessary for your chosen career?

_____

4. Research community colleges and universities in your area and plot out an educational plan to follow if you want this career.

_____

_____

_____

_____

_____

_____

_____

_____

_____

_____

_____

5. Visit the *Occupational Outlook Handbook* online to research the job outlook for this particular career. Record your findings here.

_____

_____

_____

6. According to the *Occupational Outlook Handbook*, what is a typical salary for someone in this career?

_____

7. Based on your knowledge of this career, would you consider this career in the future? Why or why not?

_____

_____

_____

_____

_____

_____

Name _____ Date _____ Period _____

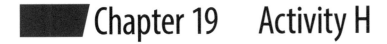 Chapter 19   Activity H

Practice Test

Completion

Instructions: *Write the term that completes the statement in the space provided.*

1. STIs can damage the reproductive organs and cause _____, the inability to conceive and have children.

   _____

2. _____ is sometimes called the *great imitator* because its symptoms resemble those of many other diseases.

   _____

3. Doctors screen for cervical cancer, which can be caused by HPV, using a(n) _____ test.

   _____

4. A latex _____ can provide a barrier against pathogens during sexual activity.

   _____

5. HIV targets immune cells called _____ cells, including T-helper cells, which activate and coordinate the immune system.

   _____

True/False

Instructions: *Indicate whether each statement below is true or false.*

6. _____ *True or false?* Engaging in sexual activity one time with just one partner who has an STI is all it takes to contract an STI.

7. _____ *True or false?* Chlamydia does *not* affect female reproductive health.

8. _____ *True or false?* Late-stage syphilis does *not* include obvious external signs.

9. _____ *True or false?* Having other STIs increases the risk of transmitting and contracting HIV.

10. _____ *True or false?* Anti-discrimination laws protect people with HIV, but not the families of people with HIV.

Multiple Choice

Instructions: *Select the letter that corresponds to the correct answer.*

11. _____ Which of the following STIs can cause dementia and paralysis if left untreated?
    A. syphilis   C. chlamydia
    B. HPV   D. trichomoniasis

12. _____ HSV type 2 causes infections on the _____.
    A. mouth   C. genitals
    B. lips   D. All of the above.

13. _____ Sexual _____ is the only method that is 100-percent effective in preventing STIs.
    A. prevention   C. treatment
    B. abstinence   D. infection

14. _____ You *cannot* reduce risk for STIs using _____.
    A. condoms   C. birth control pills
    B. abstinence   D. refusal skills

15. _____ Which of the following can transmit HIV?
   A. spit, sweat, or tears
   B. using the same toilet seat
   C. kissing or hugging
   D. injections with unsterilized needles

Matching

Instructions: *Match each key term to its definition (16–22).*

16. _____ showing few or no signs of infection or disease

17. _____ infection of the fallopian tubes and pelvic cavity that sometimes leads to infertility

18. _____ bloodborne virus that infects and kills the body's cells, weakening the immune system

19. _____ amount of HIV in the blood

20. _____ common STI that infects cells in the skin and membranes, causing them to grow abnormally

21. _____ abnormal cancerous growth of the cervix

22. _____ health condition in which the body can no longer fight infections and diseases

A. acquired immunodeficiency syndrome (AIDS)

B. asymptomatic

C. cervical cancer

D. human immunodeficiency virus (HIV)

E. human papillomavirus (HPV)

F. pelvic inflammatory disease (PID)

G. viral load

Analyzing Data

Instructions: *The following chart presents data from the Centers for Disease Control and Prevention about new STI diagnoses over recent years. Use the information provided to answer the following questions.*

STI	2015	2016	2017	2018	2019
Chlamydia	1,526,658	1,598,354	1,708,569	1,758,668	1,808,703
Gonorrhea	395,216	468,514	555,608	583,405	616,392
Syphilis	74,707	88,053	101,584	115,045	129,813

Centers for Disease Control and Prevention

Figure 2. Number of STI diagnoses by year

23. 779,367 of the chlamydia diagnoses in 2018 were among females aged 15 to 24. What percentage of the total chlamydia diagnoses is this?

_____

24. By what percent did the syphilis diagnosis rate increase from 2015 to 2019?

_____

Short Answer

Instructions: *Answer the following questions using what you have learned in this chapter.*

25. Explain the difference in treatment for bacterial STIs and viral STIs.

_____

_____

_____

26. Do people die from HIV, AIDS, or opportunistic infections associated with AIDS? Explain your answer.

_____

_____

_____

CHAPTER 20 / Noncommunicable Diseases

Lesson 20.1   Activity A

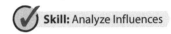
Skill: Analyze Influences

What Are the Risk Factors?

Instructions: *Read the following scenarios. Identify specific factors that may influence each individual's risk of developing a noncommunicable disease. Categorize each factor as behavioral, environmental, or genetic.*

Scenarios

1. At 65, Silvia has lived longer than her parents, who died of cancer and a stroke, did. Silvia is very proud of quitting smoking after 40 years. Her doctors warn that her high-fat diet may cause atherosclerosis, but Silvia is sure she is not at risk for any serious diseases.

   A. Identify factors that influence Silvia's risk of developing a noncommunicable disease.

   _____

   _____

2. George spends much of his time watching TV and has a sweet tooth. His partner worries about George's health, especially since he works in a factory that exposes him to hazardous chemicals.

   A. Identify factors that influence George's risk of developing a noncommunicable disease.

   _____

   _____

3. Jaime is enjoying some time off work while his office building is temporarily closed. Construction crews found asbestos in the building's insulation. Jaime has decided to spend his time off relaxing on his patio, reading a book, and smoking cigars.

   A. Identify factors that influence Jaime's risk of developing a noncommunicable disease.

   _____

   _____

4. Ben recently celebrated his 50th birthday at a steakhouse. For dinner, he had a porterhouse steak, asparagus, and a glass of red wine. Unfortunately, Ben's father was unable to attend the celebration because he was experiencing gout.

   A. Identify factors that influence Ben's risk of developing a noncommunicable disease.

   _____

   _____

Question

1. Think about your risk for noncommunicable diseases. What are your risk factors? How can you reduce this risk today and as you age?

   _____

   _____

   _____

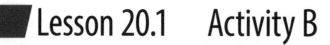 Lesson 20.1   Activity B

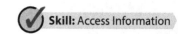

Interviewing an Adult

Instructions: *For this activity, conduct an interview with a parent or other trusted adult about noncommunicable diseases. Record responses from your interview. Make sure to thank your parent or trusted adult for agreeing to be interviewed. Then, answer the questions that follow.*

Name of Interviewee: _____

Interview Questions

1. Have you been diagnosed with a noncommunicable disease? Which disease? If not, give an example of someone you know who has.

    A. Response: _____

    _____

2. How was this disease diagnosed? (Were there signs or symptoms? Did a doctor perform a screening or physical exam?)

    A. Response: _____

    _____

3. Was the disease acute or chronic? What was the prognosis (statement about the likely outcome) for this disease?

    A. Response: _____

    _____

4. What was the treatment plan? Did the plan include changes in behavior, medications, or therapy?

    A. Response: _____

    _____

5. Did the disease go into remission? Did the disease relapse? Explain.

    A. Response: _____

    _____

6. Additional question: _____

    A. Response: _____

    _____

Questions

1. What were the most interesting things you learned?

    _____

    _____

    _____

2. How did this interview help shape the way you view and understand noncommunicable diseases? Explain.

    _____

    _____

Name _____ Date _____ Period _____

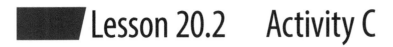 Lesson 20.2   Activity C

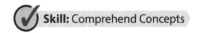 **Skill:** Comprehend Concepts

Cardiovascular Emergencies

Instructions: *Many different parts of the body can signal a medical emergency of the cardiovascular system, including heart attack, stroke, and congestive heart failure. Answer the following questions about each medical emergency.*

1. List the signs and symptoms of a heart attack associated with each body part listed.

    A. Head: _____

    B. Jaw, neck, back: _____

    C. Chest: _____

    D. Arm or shoulder: _____

    E. Lungs: _____

    F. Stomach: _____

    G. Heart: _____

2. What other symptoms might a person who is having a heart attack experience?

    _____

    _____

    _____

    _____

3. Where might someone experience numbness or weakness if experiencing a stroke?

    _____

4. What symptoms of a stroke affect a person's brain function?

    _____

    _____

    _____

    _____

5. List the signs and symptoms of congestive heart failure associated with each body part listed.

    A. Ankle: _____

    B. Lungs: _____

    C. Skin and lips: _____

6. What should you do if a person experiences symptoms of a stroke, heart attack, or congestive heart failure?

    _____

    _____

    _____

    _____

    _____

    _____

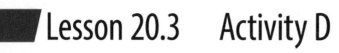 Lesson 20.3   Activity D

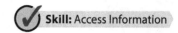 **Skill:** Access Information

Cancer Research

Instructions: *Choose one type of cancer to research to learn more about. Use at least three different reliable resources. Organize your research using the questions in this activity.*

1. Which type of cancer did you decide to research?

    _____

2. What sources did you use? List the article name, author, and sponsor organization for each.

    A. Source #1

    Name of organization: _____

    Title of article or page: _____

    Author name: _____

    B. Source #2

    Name of organization: _____

    Title of article or page: _____

    Author name: _____

    C. Source #3

    Name of organization: _____

    Title of article or page: _____

    Author name: _____

3. What are the causes and risk factors for this type of cancer?

    _____

    _____

4. What are the signs and symptoms of this type of cancer?

    _____

    _____

5. How can this type of cancer be detected? What test(s) can diagnose this disease?

    _____

    _____

6. What strategies could you use to help prevent this type of cancer?

    _____

    _____

7. How is this type of cancer typically treated?

    _____

    _____

8. What questions do you still have about this topic? (Identify at least two questions.)

    _____

    _____

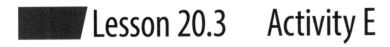 Lesson 20.3   Activity E

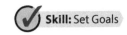

Preventing Cancer

Instructions: *Set a SMART goal to reduce risk factors and prevent yourself from developing cancer. Answer the following questions to help you achieve your objective.*

1. List at least five actions you can take that would reduce your risk for developing cancer.

   _____

   _____

   _____

   _____

   _____

   _____

   _____

2. Create a central goal to prevent cancer.

   _____

   _____

3. To be sure your goal is SMART, indicate how it meets each of the following.

   A. Specific: _____

   B. Measurable: _____

   C. Achievable: _____

   D. Relevant: _____

   E. Timely: _____

4. List three short-term goals that will help you achieve your larger goal.

   A. Goal: _____

   _____

   B. Goal: _____

   _____

   C. Goal: _____

   _____

5. Name one obstacle that might stop you from achieving your goal. How can you overcome this obstacle?

   _____

   _____

   _____

   _____

6. What people or resources can help you achieve your goal?

   _____

   _____

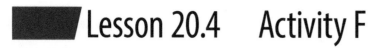 Lesson 20.4   Activity F

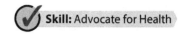 Skill: Advocate for Health

Noncommunicable Diseases

Instructions: *For each noncommunicable disease, list the health effects and risk factors. Then, create a campaign to spread this information to other students at your school.*

Noncommunicable Diseases

1. Type 2 diabetes mellitus

   A. List the health effects and symptoms. _____

   _____

   B. List the risk factors. _____

2. Alzheimer's disease

   A. List the health effects and symptoms. _____

   _____

   B. List the risk factors. _____

3. Gout

   A. List the health effects and symptoms. _____

   _____

   B. List the risk factors. _____

4. Osteoporosis

   A. List the health effects and symptoms. _____

   _____

   B. List the risk factors. _____

5. Asthma

   A. List the health effects and symptoms. _____

   _____

   B. List the risk factors. _____

Questions

1. If the target audience for your informational campaign is other students at your school, what do you think is the best medium to get the message out? Explain.

   _____

   _____

2. After you complete your campaign, reflect on how well it promoted health information to others. Would you do anything differently in future health campaigns? Why or why not?

   _____

   _____

   _____

Chapter 20   Activity G

Practice Test

Completion

Instructions: *Write the term that completes the statement in the space provided.*

1. _____ is the body's internal, steady state of balance.

   _____

2. The procedure that removes a sample of tissue from the body for testing is called a(n) _____.

   _____

3. Diabetes mellitus is a disease characterized by _____, a condition of high blood sugar.

   _____

4. Produced by the pancreas, _____ is a hormone that signals cells to move sugar from the blood into surrounding cells.

   _____

5. Allergies that affect the entire body rather than one specific organ is a(n) _____ allergy.

   _____

True/False

Instructions: *Indicate whether each statement below is true or false.*

6. _____ *True or false?* Relapse is a period of time without signs and symptoms associated with a disease.

7. _____ *True or false?* Veins are large, muscular blood vessels that carry blood from the heart to the capillaries.

8. _____ *True or false?* The aorta is the largest vein in the body.

9. _____ *True or false?* A benign tumor is *not* cancerous.

10. _____ *True or false?* Alzheimer's disease is a progressive disease, which means it grows worse over time.

Multiple Choice

Instructions: *Select the letter that corresponds to the correct answer.*

11. _____ Noncommunicable diseases develop due to _____.
   A. genes
   B. diet
   C. behaviors
   D. All of the above.

12. _____ There are two types of stroke: ischemic stroke and the less common _____.
   A. hemorrhagic stroke
   B. warning stroke
   C. transient ischemic attack
   D. ministroke

13. _____ _____ is a condition in which the heart becomes too weak to pump blood effectively.
   A. Atherosclerosis
   B. Congestive heart failure
   C. Coronary artery disease
   D. Hypertension

14. _____ Malignant tumors can _____, or spread from their original location to other parts of the body.
   A. mutate
   B. biopsy
   C. metamorphose
   D. metastasize

15. _____ Which of the following conditions is a dangerous side effect of type 1 diabetes mellitus?
   A. epilepsy
   B. anaphylaxis
   C. gout
   D. acidosis

Matching

Instructions: *Match each key term to its definition (16–22).*

16. _____ use of medications to kill cancer cells and shrink malignant tumors

17. _____ disease in which the walls of the arteries thicken, harden, and become inflexible

18. _____ procedure that uses X-rays to image the breast and screen for breast cancer

19. _____ pain in the chest that often accompanies a heart attack

20. _____ autoimmune disease in which the body's immune system attacks the joints

21. _____ disease that makes bones weak, brittle, and prone to fractures

22. _____ chemical that causes blood vessels to leak fluids into tissues

A. angina
B. arteriosclerosis
C. chemotherapy
D. histamine
E. mammogram
F. osteoporosis
G. rheumatoid arthritis

Analyzing Data

Instructions: *Use the information provided by the Centers for Disease Control and Prevention to answer the following questions.*

Leading Causes of Death in the US 2019	Deaths
Influenza and pneumonia	49,783
Diabetes	87,647
Alzheimer's disease	121,499
Stroke	150,005
Chronic lower respiratory diseases	156,979
Accidents	173,040
Cancer	599,601
Heart disease	659,041

Centers for Disease Control and Prevention

Figure 1. Leading causes of death in the US in 2019

23. What percent of the 1,997,595 deaths shown was caused by heart disease?

_____

24. How many of these leading causes of death in the US are noncommunicable diseases?

_____

25. How many more deaths are caused by cancer than by stroke?

_____

Short Answer

Instructions: *Answer the following questions using what you have learned in this chapter.*

26. How are communicable and noncommunicable diseases different?

_____

_____

27. Explain the difference between type 1 diabetes mellitus and type 2 diabetes mellitus.

_____

_____

_____

_____

CHAPTER 21 / The Beginning of Life

Lesson 21.1   Activity A   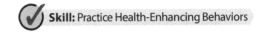 **Skill:** Practice Health-Enhancing Behaviors

The Male Reproductive System

Instructions: *Answer the following questions about the male reproductive system's anatomy and care.*

1. Which organs of the male reproductive system produce sperm and testosterone?

   _____

2. What is the name of the saclike structure that holds the testes?

   _____

3. What is the name of the tube that carries sperm from the epididymis to the penis?

   _____

4. Which structure of the male reproductive system carries urine and semen out of the body?

   _____

5. Which part of the male reproductive system contains erectile tissue?

   _____

6. What is ejaculation?

   _____

7. Explain how each of the following steps can help maintain the health of the male reproductive system.

   A. Abstain from sexual activity or use a condom: _____

   _____

   _____

   B. Practice hygiene: _____

   _____

   _____

   C. Perform testicular self-examinations: _____

   _____

   _____

   D. Visit the doctor: _____

   _____

   _____

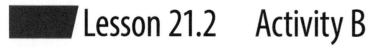 ## Lesson 21.2   Activity B

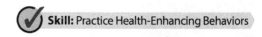 **Skill:** Practice Health-Enhancing Behaviors

The Female Reproductive System

Instructions: *Answer the following questions about the female reproductive system's anatomy and care.*

1. Which organs of the female reproductive system contain immature eggs?

   _____

2. What is the name of the structure that leads from each ovary to each side of the uterus?

   _____

3. Which organ of the female reproductive system houses a developing baby during pregnancy?

   _____

4. What is the name for the narrow passage that connects the uterus and vagina?

   _____

5. Which structure of the female reproductive system is also called the *birth canal*?

   _____

6. Which part of the female reproductive system contains erectile tissue?

   _____

7. What is the function of the mammary glands?

   _____

8. Explain how each of the following steps can help maintain the health of the female reproductive system.

   A. Abstain from sexual activity or use a condom: _____

   _____

   _____

   B. Maintain hygiene: _____

   _____

   _____

   C. Practice breast awareness: _____

   _____

   _____

   D. See a doctor: _____

   _____

   _____

Name _____ Date _____ Period _____

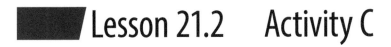 Lesson 21.2   Activity C

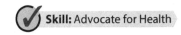

Diseases and Disorders

Instructions: *Both the male and female reproductive systems can be vulnerable to a variety of diseases and disorders. Using the information you have learned, fill in the information for each disease or disorder.*

1. Cryptorchidism

   A. Male or female? _____

   B. Definition: _____

   C. Symptoms: _____

   D. Treatments: _____

2. Endometriosis

   A. Male or female? _____

   B. Definition: _____

   C. Symptoms: _____

   D. Treatments: _____

3. Epididymitis

   A. Male or female? _____

   B. Definition: _____

   C. Symptoms: _____

   D. Treatments: _____

4. Ovarian cysts

   A. Male or female? _____

   B. Definition: _____

   C. Symptoms: _____

   D. Treatments: _____

5. Premenstrual syndrome (PMS)

   A. Male or female? _____

   B. Definition: _____

   C. Symptoms: _____

   D. Treatments: _____

6. Prostatitis

   A. Male or female? _____

   B. Definition: _____

   C. Symptoms: _____

   D. Treatments: _____

Instructions: *In small groups, create a campaign to inform teens in your community about common diseases and disorders of the reproductive systems. Use the medium of your choice to distribute your information.*

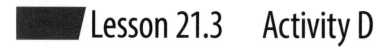 Lesson 21.3   Activity D

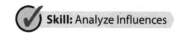

Influences on Pregnancy Health

Instructions: *Read the following scenarios and answer the questions about the influences that affect the health of a pregnancy.*

Scenario 1

At 30, Brandon and his wife are very excited for their first child. Together, they decide to start a regular physical activity routine to maintain their health throughout the pregnancy. To honor their success at maintaining this routine, Brandon and his wife each celebrate with a beer every Friday night.

1. Which behavior of Brandon's wife can negatively affect the health of her pregnancy?

_____

2. What health effect does this behavior have on the baby? Which serious health conditions might their baby develop through this behavior?

_____

_____

Scenario 2

Jasmine is 20 years old and pregnant with twins. She knows that some swelling is normal throughout pregnancy, so she was not concerned at first about the swelling in her legs, feet, and hands. She also experiences some headaches and dizziness. At a recent checkup, Jasmine's doctor tells her that she has developed preeclampsia.

1. What risk factors may have contributed to Jasmine's preeclampsia?

_____

2. How can prenatal care reduce the risk of this complication?

_____

_____

Scenario 3

Alicia was diagnosed with pelvic inflammatory disease (PID) a few years ago. She developed this disease from a chlamydia infection. She recently learned that she is pregnant and worries about how her PID might influence her pregnancy.

1. Which pregnancy complication is Alicia at risk for due to her PID?

_____

2. Describe this complication.

_____

_____

3. What can happen to Alicia's fallopian tubes due to this complication? How would this affect Alicia's health?

_____

_____

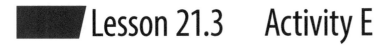 Lesson 21.3   Activity E

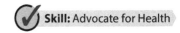 **Skill:** Advocate for Health

Create a Pregnancy Care Plan

Instructions: *Jada and Luis are expecting their first child in the spring. Unlike you, Jada and Luis never took health courses in high school, and therefore do not know what to expect for this pregnancy. For this activity, fill in the information to help Jada and Luis create a pregnancy care plan.*

Doctor's Appointments

1. Recommended frequency: _____

2. What to expect at the first appointment: _____
   _____
   _____

3. What to expect at follow-up appointments: _____
   _____
   _____

Changes to the Body

1. Physical changes: _____
   _____
   _____
   _____

2. Emotional changes: _____
   _____
   _____

3. Unpleasant side effects: _____
   _____
   _____

Nutrition and Physical Activity

1. Normal amount of weight gain: _____

2. Number of calories to add to daily diet: _____

3. Foods and substances to avoid: _____
   _____
   _____

4. Physical activity recommendations: _____
   _____
   _____

Lesson 21.4   Activity F

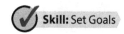

Pregnancy Prevention Goals .

Instructions: *Develop a SMART goal to prevent pregnancies throughout your teen years. Fill out the following information to build your goal.*

1. Below is a list of various contraceptive methods. Indicate each method you would feel comfortable using to prevent pregnancies.

   A. _____ Birth control implant   J. _____ Fertility awareness methods (FAM)

   B. _____ Birth control patch   K. _____ Internal condom

   C. _____ Birth control pill   L. _____ Intrauterine device (IUD)

   D. _____ Birth control shot   M._____ Sexual abstinence

   E. _____ Cervical cap   N. _____ Spermicide

   F. _____ Contraceptive sponge   O. _____ Sterilization

   G. _____ Diaphragm   P. _____ Vaginal ring

   H. _____ Emergency contraceptive pills Q. _____ Withdrawal

   I. _____ External condom

2. Review the effectiveness of various contraceptive methods. Which of the methods that you selected is the most effective? least effective?

   _____

   _____

   _____

3. Now, make a SMART goal to prevent pregnancies throughout the teen years. To be sure your goal is SMART, indicate how it meets each of the following.

   A. Specific: _____

   B. Measurable: _____

   C. Achievable: _____

   D. Relevant: _____

   E. Timely: _____

4. What interpersonal skills might you need to implement and uphold your goal? Explain.

   _____

   _____

   _____

5. What obstacles might get in your way of preventing pregnancies? How can you overcome these obstacles?

   _____

   _____

   _____

   _____

   _____

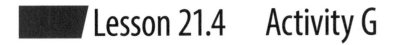 Lesson 21.4   Activity G

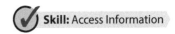 **Skill:** Access Information

Infant Care Careers

Instructions: *When choosing a healthcare career, be mindful of your personal interests, strengths, and weaknesses. These will help you decide which career would best suit you. Study the information in the chart below and answer the questions that follow. Do additional research as needed to complete the activity.*

Career	Interest/Quality	Duties	Education and Training	Resource
Pediatric nurse	Enjoys working with infants	Delivers healthcare for newborns and infants	Associate's degree or bachelor's degree	American Nurses Association
Certified nurse-midwife	Enjoys working with infants Would enjoy assisting with childbirth	Provides postnatal care Provides assistance with delivery	College degree, graduate training, certification	American College of Nurse-Midwives
Obstetrician	Enjoys working with infants Would enjoy assisting with childbirth Is interested in science	Provides postnatal care Delivers babies Diagnoses and treats conditions related to pregnancy and childbirth	Bachelor's degree, medical degree	American Medical Association, American Congress of Obstetricians and Gynecologists
Licensed practical nurse (LPN)	Enjoys working with infants Enjoys working with patients of all ages	Administers basic nursing care to all patients	High school diploma, LPN certification/license	National Federation of Licensed Practical Nurses
Pediatrician	Enjoys working with patients of all ages Patience Good communication skills	Provides care for infants, children, teens, and young adults Administers vaccines and treats common illnesses, minor injuries, and infectious diseases	Bachelor's degree, medical degree, residency experience	American Academy of Pediatrics
Neonatal nurse	Enjoys working with infants Good communication skills Enjoys working in a fast-paced environment	Cares for babies, often premature infants, in a hospital's neonatal intensive care unit (NICU) Works directly with parents to provide education and comfort	RN or LPN certification, certification in neonatal resuscitation or neonatal intensive care	National Association of Neonatal Nurses, Academy of Neonatal Nursing

Figure 1. Information about infant care careers

1. Which of these careers most interests you? Explain why you think this career suits your interests and personal qualities.

_____

_____

_____

_____

_____

2. Research this career further. Visit the resource listed in the chart and compose a "day in the life" for someone with that career. Does this type of workday sound interesting to you?

_____

_____

_____

_____

_____

3. According to the chart, what level of education is necessary for your chosen career?

_____

4. Research community colleges and universities in your area and plot out an educational plan to follow if you want this career.

_____

_____

_____

_____

_____

_____

_____

_____

_____

_____

_____

_____

_____

_____

_____

5. Visit the *Occupational Outlook Handbook* online to research the job outlook for this particular career. Record your findings here.

_____

_____

_____

6. According to the *Occupational Outlook Handbook*, what is a typical salary for someone in this career?

_____

7. Based on your knowledge of this career, would you consider this career in the future? Why or why not?

_____

_____

_____

_____

_____

◢ Chapter 21 Activity H

Practice Test

Completion

Instructions: *Write the term that completes the statement in the space provided.*

1. During the teen years, males should perform _____ self-examinations to watch for signs of cancer and hernia.

   _____

2. The _____ is a hollow, muscular organ of the female reproductive system that houses a developing baby until it is born.

   _____

3. A female's first menstrual cycle, or _____, generally occurs between 10 and 15 years of age.

   _____

4. Development that happens during gestation is called _____ development.

   _____

5. _____ laws allow people to leave their babies at certain facilities with no questions asked and no legal consequences.

   _____

True/False

Instructions: *Indicate whether each statement below is true or false.*

6. _____ *True or false?* Semen is another name for sperm.

7. _____ *True or false?* Pelvic inflammatory disease (PID) is a preventable condition often caused by STIs.

8. _____ *True or false?* Recessive genes always cause certain characteristics in a child.

9. _____ *True or false?* The lungs and liver are the last organs to complete fetal development.

10. _____ *True or false?* Legal fatherhood establishes the male parent's right to be the custodial parent for all children.

Multiple Choice

Instructions: *Select the letter that corresponds to the correct answer.*

11. _____ Which of the following parts of the male reproductive system is responsible for secreting fluid that mixes with sperm to form semen?
    A. vas deferens
    B. testis
    C. bulbourethral gland
    D. prostate

12. _____ The _____ serves as the birth canal.
    A. uterus
    B. fallopian tube
    C. vagina
    D. labia

13. _____ _____ is a pregnancy complication characterized by high blood pressure.
    A. Gestational diabetes mellitus
    B. Miscarriage
    C. Preeclampsia
    D. Ectopic pregnancy

14. _____ The _____ is a fertilized egg implanted in the uterus.
    A. embryo
    B. chorion
    C. blastocyst
    D. amnion

15. _____ Which of the following describes an adoption in which adopted children may have contact with their biological parents?

    A. visiting adoption   C. closed adoption

    B. open adoption   D. temporary adoption

Matching

Instructions: *Match each key term to its definition (16–22).*

16. _____ condition in which uterine tissue grows outside the uterus

17. _____ noncancerous tumors of the uterus

18. _____ noncancerous tumors on the ovaries

19. _____ lengthening and hardening of the penis due to sexual stimulation

20. _____ tube that carries sperm from the epididymis to the penis

21. _____ release of a mature egg from one of the ovarian follicles

22. _____ mass of erectile tissue that swells and enlarges during sexual arousal

A. clitoris

B. endometriosis

C. erection

D. fibroids

E. ovarian cysts

F. ovulation

G. vas deferens

Analyzing Data

Instructions: *The table below shows the live birth rates per 1,000 US females, ages 15–19, between 2007 and 2019 according to the National Center for Health Statistics division of the CDC. Use the information provided to answer the following questions.*

Year	2007	2012	2019
Total	41.5	29.4	16.7
Hispanic	75.3	46.3	25.3
White	27.2	20.5	11.4
Black	62.0	43.9	25.8
Asian	13.4	8.5	2.7
American Indian or Alaska Native	66.3	51.2	29.2

National Center for Health Statistics

Figure 2. Live births per 1,000 females, ages 15 to 19

23. What percentage of Hispanic females aged 15–19 had a live birth in 2007? in 2019? _____

24. Describe the general trend among live births for females aged 15–19.

_____

Short Answer

Instructions: *Answer the following questions using what you have learned in this chapter.*

25. List the three stages of prenatal development and explain when each stage begins and ends.

_____

_____

_____

26. Explain some of the physical challenges of teen parenthood for the parent and the child.

_____

_____

_____

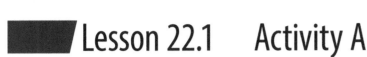

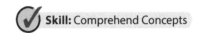

Lesson 22.1   Activity A

Skill: Comprehend Concepts

The Human Life Cycle

Instructions: *For each of the developmental stages, identify the age range associated with that stage and describe the typical developments associated with that stage. Include descriptions of physical, intellectual, emotional, and social development across the life span. Compare your responses with classmates.*

Stage: Early Childhood

1. Age range: _____

2. Development: _____

_____

_____

Stage: Middle Childhood

1. Age range: _____

2. Development: _____

_____

_____

Stage: Adolescence

1. Age range: _____

2. Development: _____

_____

_____

Stage: Adulthood

1. Age range: _____

2. Development: _____

_____

_____

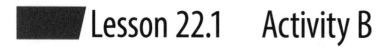 Lesson 22.1   Activity B

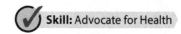 Skill: Advocate for Health

Promoting Respect

Instructions: *Read the following scenarios and explain how you can respond to each situation in a way that promotes respect of the developmental differences of each individual.*

Scenario 1

Antonio is in your class at school. He has an autism spectrum disorder that sometimes makes social interactions difficult for him. Some of your other classmates like to make fun of the way Antonio communicates, even mocking him when he tries to talk to them.

1. How can you and your friends intervene on Antonio's behalf?

_____

_____

_____

2. In what ways can your school community promote respect for people with developmental differences?

_____

_____

_____

Scenario 2

Cameron had his legs amputated due to a military injury. He now uses a wheelchair to get most places. Cameron loves working at the library, and they make sure he has the accommodations he needs to do his job, including automatic doors, ramps, and elevators. He takes the bus to work each day, which is also accessible for him.

1. What law ensures that Cameron has the same rights as people without physical disabilities? In what ways does this law affect Cameron's daily life?

_____

_____

_____

Scenario 3

Angela finds mathematics incredibly frustrating. She does not understand how people can calculate equations so easily. She always gets her numbers out of order. Angela feels embarrassed about how difficult math is for her, so she tends to not ask questions when she is confused.

1. What learning disorder does Angela likely have?

_____

2. How can teachers, classmates, and family members support Angela?

_____

_____

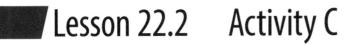 Lesson 22.2   Activity C

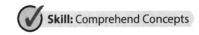 **Skill:** Comprehend Concepts

The Childhood Years

Instructions: *For each of the scenarios, identify the individual's stage of life (infancy, toddler years, preschool years, or middle childhood) and identify what type of development is taking place: physical, social, emotional, or intellectual.*

1. Joey plays soccer with his sister in the backyard all the time. He is the best player on his soccer team.

    A. What is Joey's stage of life? _____

    B. What type of development is taking place? Explain. _____

    _____

2. Casey realizes that shaking her rattle causes it to make a noise.

    A. What is Casey's stage of life? _____

    B. What type of development is taking place? Explain. _____

    _____

3. Bradley watches other children play in the park and enjoys playing on his own nearby.

    A. What is Bradley's stage of life? _____

    B. What type of development is taking place? Explain. _____

    _____

4. Jhumpa forms a strong attachment to her mother as her mother talks and laughs with her.

    A. What is Jhumpa's stage of life?_____

    B. What type of development is taking place? Explain. _____

    _____

5. Elijah uses child safety scissors to cut up colorful paper.

    A. What is Elijah's stage of life? _____

    B. What type of development is taking place? Explain. _____

    _____

6. A girl in Tiana's class invited her to a sleepover. Tiana is excited to make a new friend.

    A. What is Tiana's stage of life?_____

    B. What type of development is taking place? Explain. _____

    _____

7. Devin still mispronounces or forgets some words, but loves to retell stories he reads.

    A. What is Devin's stage of life? _____

    B. What type of development is taking place? Explain. _____

    _____

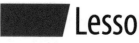 Lesson 22.2   Activity D

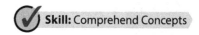

Development During Childhood

Instructions: *During early and middle childhood, important growth and development takes place. For each of the following stages of life, write a short story about a child that indicates at least one form of social, emotional, intellectual, and physical development each.*

Infancy

1. Write a story.

_____

_____

_____

_____

_____

Toddler Years

1. Write a story.

_____

_____

_____

_____

_____

Preschool Years

1. Write a story.

_____

_____

_____

_____

_____

Middle Childhood

1. Write a story.

_____

_____

_____

_____

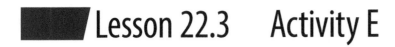   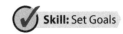

Lesson 22.3   Activity E

Handling Health and Wellness Issues

Instructions: *With a partner, choose one of the skills for handling adolescent health and wellness issues in the text. Together, brainstorm a SMART goal you could set to use this skill. Act on this SMART goal, and hold each other accountable.*

1. Health and wellness skill chosen: _____

2. Create a central goal to use this skill.

   _____

   _____

   _____

3. To be sure your goal is SMART, indicate how it meets each of the following.

   A. Specific: _____

   B. Measurable: _____

   C. Achievable: _____

   D. Relevant: _____

   E. Timely: _____

4. List three short-term goals that will help you on your way to achieving your larger goal.

   A. Goal: _____

   _____

   B. Goal: _____

   _____

   C. Goal: _____

   _____

5. How will you monitor your progress?

   _____

   _____

   _____

6. How can you help keep your partner on track? How can you and your partner stay accountable for your own actions?

   _____

   _____

   _____

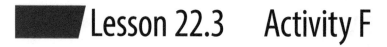 Lesson 22.3   Activity F

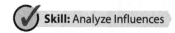 **Skill:** Analyze Influences

The Influence of Adolescence

Instructions: *Describe how each of the following statements about adolescence can be both a positive and a negative influence on teen health and development.*

1. An adolescent's brain is more developed than it was in childhood, but in many ways will continue to develop into young adulthood.

   A. How can this be a positive influence on teen health and development?

   _____

   _____

   _____

   _____

   B. How can this be a negative influence on teen health and development?

   _____

   _____

   _____

   _____

2. During adolescence, a person's social world expands beyond the family and even close friends. The need to feel accepted becomes increasingly important.

   A. How can this be a positive influence on teen health and development?

   _____

   _____

   _____

   _____

   B. How can this be a negative influence on teen health and development?

   _____

   _____

   _____

   _____

3. Adolescents experience increases in school activities, friendships, and work opportunities.

   A. How can this be a positive influence on teen health and development?

   _____

   _____

   _____

   _____

   B. How can this be a negative influence on teen health and development?

   _____

   _____

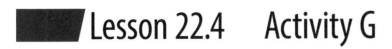 **Lesson 22.4   Activity G**

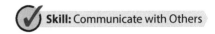

Understanding Adulthood

Instructions: *People continue to change and develop throughout adulthood. Interview someone who fits into each stage of adulthood—young, middle, and older adulthood. Ask each interviewee the questions provided, and record their answers here. Make sure you use active listening skills and communicate respectfully with each adult.*

Young Adulthood

1. List the interviewee's information.

   A. Name: _____

   B. Age: _____

   C. Relationship to you: _____

2. Since there is no "typical" young adult in the United States, what is your definition of young adulthood?

   _____

   _____

   _____

   _____

3. What has been the biggest change in your life from adolescence to young adulthood?

   _____

   _____

   _____

   _____

4. What personal goals are you working toward in young adulthood?

   _____

   _____

   _____

   _____

Middle Adulthood

1. List the interviewee's information.

   A. Name: _____

   B. Age: _____

   C. Relationship to you: _____

2. Were you worried about entering middle adulthood? Were those worries valid?

   _____

   _____

   _____

   _____

3. What has surprised you the most about middle adulthood?

_____

_____

_____

_____

4. What are some of your greatest achievements during middle adulthood?

_____

_____

_____

_____

Older Adulthood

1. List the interviewee's information.

   A. Name: _____

   B. Age: _____

   C. Relationship to you: _____

2. What do you spend most of your time doing?

_____

_____

_____

_____

3. What is the greatest source of happiness in your life at this time?

_____

_____

_____

_____

4. What advice would you give to a teen about to enter adulthood?

_____

_____

_____

_____

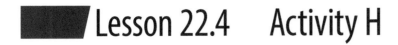 Lesson 22.4   Activity H

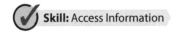 Skill: Access Information

Older Adult Care Careers

Instructions: *When choosing a healthcare career, be mindful of your personal interests, strengths, and weaknesses. These will help you decide which career would best suit you. Study the information in the chart below and answer the questions that follow. Do additional research as needed to complete the activity.*

Career	Interest/Quality	Duties	Education and Training	Resource
Recreational therapist	Communication and listening skills Wants to assist with physical issues	Plans, directs, and coordinates recreational activities for older adults	Bachelor's degree and certification	American Therapeutic Recreation Association
Geriatric social worker	Communication and listening skills Wants to assist with social and emotional issues	Helps older adults solve problems Helps older adults obtain medical, psychological, and financial assistance	Master's degree	National Association of Social Workers
Nursing assistant or orderly	Enjoys working in a hospital setting Wants to assist with physical issues	Provides basic care and assistance for activities of daily living Works in hospitals or nursing homes	State-approved education program and competency exam, on-the-job training	National Association of Health Care Assistants
Rehabilitation counselor	Wants to assist with social and emotional issues Wants to assist with physical issues	Assists older adults with emotional and physical issues associated with recovery from disabilities and diseases	Master's degree and state license	American Rehabilitation Counseling Association

Figure 1. Information about older adult careers

1. Which of these careers most interests you? Explain why you think this career suits your interests and personal qualities.

_____

_____

_____

_____

_____

_____

_____

_____

_____

_____

2. Research this career further. Visit the resource listed in the chart and compose a "day in the life" for someone with that career. Does this type of workday sound interesting to you?

_____

_____

_____

_____

_____

3. According to the chart, what level of education is necessary for your chosen career?

_____

4. Research community colleges and universities in your area and plot out an educational plan to follow if you want this career.

_____

_____

_____

_____

_____

_____

_____

_____

_____

_____

_____

_____

_____

5. Visit the *Occupational Outlook Handbook* online to research the job outlook for this particular career. Record your findings here.

_____

_____

_____

_____

6. According to the *Occupational Outlook Handbook*, what is a typical salary for someone in this career?

_____

7. Based on your knowledge of this career, would you consider this career in the future? Why or why not?

_____

_____

_____

_____

_____

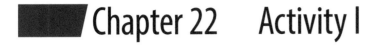 Chapter 22   Activity I

Practice Test

Completion

Instructions: *Write the term that completes the statement in the space provided.*

1. A person with a(n) _____ disability may have difficulties with learning, social behavior, communication, and self-care habits.

   _____

2. Preschoolers show rapid development of _____ skills, which involve movements that use the large muscles of the body.

   _____

3. _____ sexual characteristics include features other than reproductive organs that appear during puberty, including body hair, a deep voice, or breasts.

   _____

4. The term _____ generation describes adults who care for their aging parents as well as their own children.

   _____

5. The goal of _____ care is to bring comfort at the end of a person's life.

   _____

True/False

Instructions: *Indicate whether each statement below is true or false.*

6. _____ *True or false?* Some people reach developmental milestones earlier or later than their peers.

7. _____ *True or false?* Toddlers engage in cooperative play rather than parallel play.

8. _____ *True or false?* In females, the first sign of puberty typically occurs between 10 and 16 years of age.

9. _____ *True or false?* As muscles controlling urination weaken with age, older adults may experience incontinence.

10. _____ *True or false?* Loss of appetite, crying and feelings of sadness, and anger can all be forms of grief.

Multiple Choice

Instructions: *Select the letter that corresponds to the correct answer.*

11. _____ Which of the following is *not* a developmental stage in the human life cycle?
    A. adulthood   C. early childhood
    B. puberty   D. middle childhood

12. _____ As they improve their _____ skills, preschoolers develop the ability to draw, as well as dress and feed themselves.
    A. gross-motor   C. cooperative
    B. classification   D. fine-motor

13. _____ Puberty begins in males with enlargement of the _____.
    A. penis and testes   C. shoulders and chest
    B. arms and legs   D. muscles

14. _____ Which of the following life stages typically functions as a *sandwich generation*?
    A. adolescence   C. middle adulthood
    B. young adulthood   D. older adulthood

Matching

Instructions: *Match each key term to its definition (15–21).*

15. _____ series of developmental stages from birth through adulthood and death

16. _____ physical changes that occur as the body's reproductive system matures

17. _____ release of semen during the night while a male is sleeping

18. _____ episode of emotional upset; often includes yelling, crying, hitting, kicking, or biting

19. _____ complex, long-term disabilities that develop before adulthood and affect physical development, intellectual development, or both

20. _____ period during which egg production stops and estrogen levels drop in females

21. _____ self-directing freedom

A. autonomy

B. developmental disabilities

C. human life cycle

D. menopause

E. nocturnal emissions

F. puberty

G. temper tantrum

Analyzing Data

Instructions: *The table below illustrates information from the US Department of Education's Office of Special Education Programs about the students ages 3–21 served under the Individuals with Disabilities Education Act (IDEA) during the 2018–19 school year. Use the data to answer the questions that follow.*

Disability Type	Percentage of Students Ages 3–21 Served
Specific learning disability	33
Speech or language impairment	19
Other health impairment	15
Autism	11
Developmental delay	7
Intellectual disability	6
Emotional disturbance	5
Multiple disabilities	2
Hearing impairment	1
Orthopedic impairment	1

Office of Special Education Programs

Figure 2. Percentage of students ages 3 through 21 served under IDEA by disability

22. Which type of disability was most frequently served under IDEA in the 2018–19 school year?

_____

23. IDEA served seven million students in the 2018–19 school year. How many of these students were served for an intellectual disability?

_____

Short Answer

Instructions: *Answer the following questions using what you have learned in this chapter.*

24. What does it mean that physical, emotional, intellectual, and social development are interdependent?

_____

_____

25. Explain the role of a durable power of attorney.

_____

_____

CHAPTER 23 / Understanding Sexuality

Lesson 23.1   Activity A

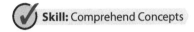 **Skill:** Comprehend Concepts

Understanding Different Types of Sexuality

Instructions: *Understanding sexuality is an important part of knowing, learning about, and accepting yourself and others. Read the following scenarios and indicate which aspect of sexuality is described (biological sex, gender identity, or sexual orientation) and the name used for and description of this personal identity.*

1. Alonso is physically attracted to both boys and girls. To try to fit in at school, he only dates girls and secretly hides his attraction for boys.

   A. Aspect of sexuality: _____

   B. Name and description of personal identity: _____

   _____

   _____

2. As a high school student, Connor is still very insecure about his genitals. He was born with an underdeveloped penis that resembled a vagina.

   A. Aspect of sexuality: _____

   B. Name and description of personal identity: _____

   _____

   _____

3. Growing up, Liu thought that because she was not attracted to boys, she might be attracted to girls instead. She has never felt attracted to girls either, however.

   A. Aspect of sexuality: _____

   B. Name and description of personal identity: _____

   _____

   _____

4. Zoe was raised female but never felt like she belonged in a female body. Within the past year, Zoe has requested to be called Bryce and identifies as a male. As Bryce, he is very happy.

   A. Aspect of sexuality: _____

   B. Name and description of personal identity: _____

   _____

   _____

5. While not yet ready to date, Hassan knows he wants to form an emotional connection and intimate relationship with a girl one day. Currently, he has crushes on some female celebrities.

   A. Aspect of sexuality: _____

   B. Name and description of personal identity: _____

   _____

   _____

6. Some days, Taylor feels like a boy, and other days, Taylor feels like a girl. Taylor's parents have been supportive and helped them find clothes that make them feel comfortable on any given day.

   A. Aspect of sexuality: _____

   B. Name and description of personal identity: _____

   _____

   _____

7. Seventeen years ago, Matt was born male. As a high school boy, Matt looks forward to his future as a man. He cannot wait to get married, find a job, have children, and travel the world.

   A. Aspect of sexuality: _____

   B. Name and description of personal identity: _____

   _____

   _____

8. Hailey used to identify as bisexual. Recently, she began dating a nonbinary person, who does not identify as a boy or a girl, and Hailey wonders if "bisexual" is a description that no longer quite fits.

   A. Aspect of sexuality: _____

   B. Name and description of personal identity: _____

   _____

   _____

9. Jordan questioned their sexuality for a long time. Jordan never really felt like a boy *or* a girl. Eventually, Jordan came to the conclusion that they did not conform to traditional gender categories.

   A. Aspect of sexuality: _____

   B. Name and description of personal identity: _____

   _____

   _____

10. Destiny has been emotionally and romantically interested in girls for the past two years. She recently started dating Sydney three months ago.

   A. Aspect of sexuality: _____

   B. Name and description of personal identity: _____

   _____

   _____

Name _____ Date _____ Period _____

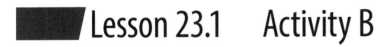 Lesson 23.1   Activity B

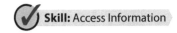

Researching Sexuality

Instructions: *Attitudes toward sexuality and gender have changed dramatically over the years. Choose a topic related to sexuality. Examples of topics might be masculinity and femininity, sexual orientation, homophobia, or disorders of sex development. Research your chosen topic using reliable online sources and then answer the following questions.*

1. How is your topic discussed and treated by society today? What are some of the opinions surrounding your topic?

    _____

    _____

    _____

    _____

    _____

2. How has this topic's treatment in society changed over the past 50 years?

    _____

    _____

    _____

    _____

3. If there has been a change, what caused it? If there has not been a change, what do you think might help cause one?

    _____

    _____

    _____

    _____

4. How do you expect treatment of this topic to change in the next 50 years?

    _____

    _____

    _____

    _____

5. Write a short reflection about the topic you chose and your research findings.

    _____

    _____

    _____

    _____

    _____

    _____

    _____

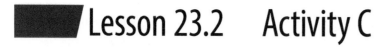 Lesson 23.2   Activity C

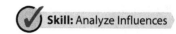

Sex in the Media

Instructions: *Sexual activity can introduce intense emotions and stress into romantic teen relationships. Unfortunately, the portrayal of sex in the media rarely considers these consequences. Watch three different teen shows or movies and pay attention to portrayals of sexual relationships. Record your observations in the spaces provided. Then, answer the questions that follow.*

1. Show or movie #1: _____

   A. Are people sexually objectified? Explain.

   _____

   _____

   _____

   B. How important are kissing and sexual activity to the story or plot?

   _____

   _____

   _____

   C. Are abstinence and birth control use discussed, shown, or implied? If so, how are these topics treated?

   _____

   _____

   _____

   _____

   D. What, if any, consequences of sexual activity are shown?

   _____

   _____

2. Show or movie #2: _____

   A. Are people sexually objectified? Explain.

   _____

   _____

   _____

   B. How important are kissing and sexual activity to the story or plot?

   _____

   _____

   _____

   C. Are abstinence and birth control use discussed, shown, or implied? If so, how are these topics treated?

   _____

   _____

   _____

   _____

D. What, if any, consequences of sexual activity are shown?

_____

_____

3. Show or movie #3: _____

A. Are people sexually objectified? Explain.

_____

_____

_____

B. How important are kissing and sexual activity to the story or plot?

_____

_____

_____

C. Are abstinence and birth control use discussed, shown, or implied? If so, how are these topics treated?

_____

_____

_____

_____

D. What, if any, consequences of sexual activity are shown?

_____

_____

Questions

1. How did the three shows or movies you watched portray teen dating relationships?

_____

_____

_____

2. Do you think that these shows portray healthy romantic or sexual relationships? Provide details.

_____

_____

_____

_____

_____

3. Do you think these shows or movies would have a positive or negative influence on the development of teen sexuality? How could their portrayal of sexual relationships impact teens watching?

_____

_____

_____

_____

4. Were the consequences of sexual activity shown or discussed in any of the shows that you watched? Provide examples.

_____

_____

_____

_____

5. Given that teens watch a fair number of movies and shows, how important do you think it is for media to portray realistic relationships that include consequences?

_____

_____

_____

6. What changes could be made in media, particularly media targeted to a teen audience, to display a more complete picture of sexuality and gender roles?

_____

_____

_____

_____

_____

_____

_____

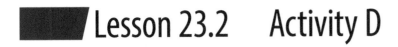 Lesson 23.2   Activity D

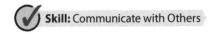

Making Sexual Decisions Together

Instructions: *Following the outline provided, role-play with a partner about how a teen couple can communicate openly about sex to make healthy decisions. In this hypothetical scenario, one partner should play a teen who is ready to engage in sexual activity. The other partner should play a teen who does not want to be sexually active.*

Discuss

1. Explain your views on sex. Include how you feel about sexual activity, why, and how you would like to prevent and handle STIs and pregnancy. Prepare your dialogue for the role-play below.

_____

_____

_____

_____

_____

_____

2. During the role-play, take notes here on your partner's views on sex.

_____

_____

_____

_____

Respect

1. Brainstorm with your partner how you can indicate to one another that you respect each other's views on sex. Note a few options below.

_____

_____

_____

_____

Agree

1. Choose a method for carrying out your mutual decision about sex. How will you stick to your decision? How will you maintain your health and safety together?

_____

_____

_____

_____

Share

1. Share information with one another about your sexual histories. Write your dialogue below.

_____

_____

_____

_____

2. Take notes on your partner's dialogue below.

_____

_____

_____

_____

3. Do either of you have any risk of STIs? How will you approach treatment or preventing transmission?

_____

_____

_____

_____

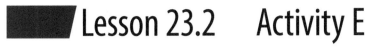 Lesson 23.2   Activity E   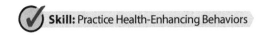 **Skill:** Practice Health-Enhancing Behaviors

What Would You Do and Say?

Instructions: *Abstinence is the best choice teens can make regarding sexual activity. Imagine you are choosing to date but remain abstinent. Refer to the textbook for guidance in remaining abstinent in a relationship. Read the following scenarios and consider what you would do and say to remain abstinent.*

1. Your partner sends you the following text: "Come over. I have a surprise for you." You drive over to find that the surprise is that your partner's parents are not home and you have the house to yourselves. Your partner has dimmed the lights and lit candles.

   A. What would you do?

   _____

   _____

   _____

   B. What would you say?

   _____

   _____

   _____

2. Your crush invites you to a party this weekend. Once there, your crush discloses wanting to have sex with you. When you explain that you would not do that, your crush says, "Wow, maybe you need to loosen up. Here, have a beer."

   A. What would you do?

   _____

   _____

   _____

   B. What would you say?

   _____

   _____

   _____

3. You are excited about going to prom, but you know the expectation about sexual activity that weekend, and you are not interested in doing those things. Your date asks if your whole friend group can get hotel rooms after prom.

   A. What would you do?

   _____

   _____

   _____

   B. What would you say?

   _____

   _____

   _____

4. You have been dating your partner for three years, and you love one another. Your partner has expressed wanting to be sexually intimate with you, but you do not feel comfortable with that. Your partner says, "I would do anything for you. Why won't you do this for me?"

A. What would you do?

_____

_____

_____

B. What would you say?

_____

_____

_____

5. You have decided to remain abstinent because the chances of an unplanned pregnancy are too great. Your new dating partner says, "How many people do you know who have gotten pregnant? It's not that big of a deal."

A. What would you do?

_____

_____

_____

B. What would you say?

_____

_____

_____

Chapter 23   Activity F

Practice Test

Completion

Instructions: *Write the term that completes the statement in the space provided.*

1. The term gender _____ refers to the unrealistic idea that the genders of man and woman are entirely opposite.

   _____

2. People who identify with a gender that does not match their biological sex are called gender _____.

   _____

3. _____ is a common abbreviation used to identify people who are nonheterosexual and/or gender nonconforming.

   _____

4. _____ are designed to help people in the LGBT+ community feel welcome, accepted, and able to discuss LGBT+ issues openly.

   _____

5. The human _____ cycle defines the physical changes that occur in the body in response to sexual arousal and activity.

   _____

True/False

Instructions: *Indicate whether each statement below is true or false.*

6. _____ *True or false?* Biological sex is more complicated than a person's sexual anatomy or sex chromosomes.

7. _____ *True or false?* Only males show their sexual excitement physically.

8. _____ *True or false?* Most sexual relationships portrayed in the media are realistic and representative of most couples.

9. _____ *True or false?* Sexual activity in teen relationships can complicate teens' emotional lives.

Multiple Choice

Instructions: *Select the letter that corresponds to the correct answer.*

10. _____ Babies with _____ syndrome have one X chromosome from one parent and no sex chromosome from the other.
    A. XO   C. Biological
    B. Turner   D. Klinefelter

11. _____ The term _____ describes the process of telling family members, friends, and others about sexual orientation or gender identity.
    A. coming out   C. identifying
    B. assigning   D. supporting

12. _____ Which of the following is *not* a phase in the human sexual response cycle?
    A. attraction   C. excitement
    B. orgasmic   D. resolution

13. _____ Families and cultures may have differing perspectives on the appropriate _____ for sexual activity.
    A. age   C. roles
    B. context   D. All of the above.

Matching

Instructions: *Match each key term to its definition (14–19).*

14. _____ hostility, anger, exclusion, and violence directed at people who are LGBT+

15. _____ element of identity that includes a person's biological sex, gender identity and expression, sexual orientation, and sexual experiences and thoughts

16. _____ enduring pattern of a person's romantic and/or sexual attraction to other people

17. _____ self-stimulation of the reproductive organs in response to sexual excitement

18. _____ identifying with the gender associated with one's biological sex

19. _____ climax of sexual excitement characterized by pleasurable muscular contractions in the reproductive organs throughout the body

A. cisgender
B. homophobia
C. masturbation
D. orgasm
E. sexual orientation
F. sexuality

Analyzing Data

Instructions: *The table below illustrates data from the 2019 Youth Risk Behavior Survey. Study the data in this table and then answer the questions that follow.*

Type of Violence	All Students	Students Who Identify as Gay, Lesbian, or Bisexual
Threatened or injured with a weapon on school property	7.4%	11.9%
Bullied on school property	19.5%	32.0%
Missed school because of safety concerns	8.7%	13.5%
Cyberbullied	15.7%	26.6%
Experienced sexual dating violence*	8.2%	16.4%
Experienced physical dating violence*	8.2%	13.1%
Forced to have sexual intercourse	7.3%	19.4%

*Among students who had dated or went out with someone during the past year

Centers for Disease Control and Prevention

Figure 1. Percentage of types of violence experienced by all students, and by students who identify as gay, lesbian, or bisexual

20. What percentage more of LGBT+ students missed school in 2019 than total students? What effect might this have on academic success?

_____

21. Why do you think LGBT+ students experience more violence than other students do?

_____

_____

Short Answer

Instructions: *Answer the following questions using what you have learned in this chapter.*

22. What are society's perceptions of the gender binary? How do you think these perceptions will change in five years? In 10 years?

_____

_____

23. Why might teens who are LGBT+ hide their sexual orientations or gender identities? How can your school environment be safer for teens who are LGBT+?

_____

_____

Name _____ Date _____ Period _____

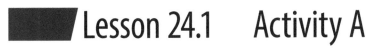 Lesson 24.1   Activity A   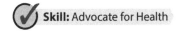 **Skill:** Advocate for Health

Practicing Abstinence

Instructions: *Imagine you are the host of an abstinence support podcast. Read each of the following requests for advice from your teen listeners. Offer strategies and advice to help your listeners maintain their commitments to abstinence. Write your dialogue in the space below and practice saying your responses aloud.*

Advice Submission 1

> Hi! My name is Tadashi, and I have been dating my girlfriend Leah for over a year now. I know some of my friends are sexually active, but I don't feel ready for sex. I think Leah feels the same way, but it's hard to be sure.

1. Write your response to Tadashi.

_____

_____

_____

_____

_____

_____

Advice Submission 2

> I've had a crush on this guy named Jamal since middle school, and we just started dating. I'm so excited that he finally is showing interest in me. The problem is that Jamal seems to want to move pretty fast, sexually, and he is my first boyfriend. I'm not really ready to go there yet, but I'm worried Jamal will dump me if I tell him that.
>
> —Jenna

1. Write your response to Jenna.

_____

_____

_____

_____

_____

_____

Advice Submission 3

My name is Carsen, and I just started dating this guy named Scott. He's a few years older than me, and I think he might not be a virgin. I'm worried that Scott will want to have a sexual relationship. If he has been sexually active, I'm also worried he may have been exposed to STIs. I'm a virgin and I know I'm not ready for sex.

1. Write your response to Carsen.

_____

_____

_____

_____

_____

_____

Advice Submission 4

Hey, quick question! Last weekend, my girlfriend, Tia, asked me what I thought about starting a sexual relationship. I told her that I was unsure about taking our relationship to that level, but I said I would think about it. Now, Tia has planned a romantic date for Friday night, and I'm worried she will make a move. I'm not sure I am ready for sex. What should I do?

From, Mario

1. Write your response to Mario.

_____

_____

_____

_____

_____

_____

Name _____ Date _____ Period _____

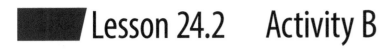 Lesson 24.2   Activity B

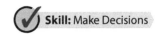

Barrier Methods

Instructions: *Listed below are some of the barrier methods for contraception. Using what you learned in your textbook, fill in the missing information. Explain why selecting each method may be a healthy decision for someone.*

1. Cervical cap

    A. Effectiveness rate: _____

    B. Estimated cost: _____

    C. How accessible is this method? Is it easy to use?

    _____

    _____

    D. Why might choosing this method be a healthy decision for someone?

    _____

    _____

    _____

2. Contraceptive sponge

    A. Effectiveness rate: _____

    B. Estimated cost: _____

    C. How accessible is this method? Is it easy to use?

    _____

    _____

    D. Why might choosing this method be a healthy decision for someone?

    _____

    _____

    _____

3. Diaphragm

    A. Effectiveness rate: _____

    B. Estimated cost: _____

    C. How accessible is this method? Is it easy to use?

    _____

    _____

    D. Why might choosing this method be a healthy decision for someone?

    _____

    _____

    _____

4. External condom

   A. Effectiveness rate: _____

   B. Estimated cost: _____

   C. How accessible is this method? Is it easy to use?

   _____

   _____

   D. Why might choosing this method be a healthy decision for someone?

   _____

   _____

   _____

5. Internal condom

   A. Effectiveness rate: _____

   B. Estimated cost: _____

   C. How accessible is this method? Is it easy to use?

   _____

   _____

   D. Why might choosing this method be a healthy decision for someone?

   _____

   _____

   _____

6. Spermicide

   A. Effectiveness rate: _____

   B. Estimated cost: _____

   C. How accessible is this method? Is it easy to use?

   _____

   _____

   D. Why might choosing this method be a healthy decision for someone?

   _____

   _____

   _____

Name _____ Date _____ Period _____

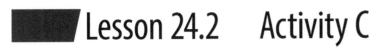 Lesson 24.2   Activity C

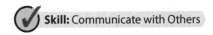

Talking About Condoms

Instructions: *Read the following pressure lines about having sex without a condom. In the space provided, indicate how you or other teens can respond to the pressure to have sex without a condom by respectfully and assertively saying no.*

1. "I don't like the way condoms feel. Let's not use them anymore."
   A. How could you respond?

   _____

   _____

   _____

2. "Let's not use a condom tonight. They kill the mood."
   A. How could you respond?

   _____

   _____

   _____

3. "I forgot to buy a condom. Not using one just this once isn't that big of a deal."
   A. How could you respond?

   _____

   _____

   _____

4. "Condoms are for people who don't trust each other. We are together and trust each other, so why do we have to use them?"
   A. How could you respond?

   _____

   _____

   _____

5. "We didn't use a condom last time and I didn't get pregnant. Let's not use one this time."
   A. How could you respond?

   _____

   _____

   _____

6. "Condoms are tight and really uncomfortable. I don't want to use them because they hurt me."
   A. How could you respond?

   _____

   _____

   _____

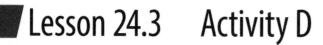 Lesson 24.3   Activity D

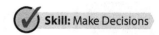

Hormonal Methods

Instructions: *Listed below are some of the hormonal methods for contraception. Using what you learned in your textbook, fill in the missing information. Explain why selecting each method may be a healthy decision for someone.*

1. Birth control implant

    A. Effectiveness rate: _____

    B. Estimated cost: _____

    C. How accessible is this method? Is it easy to use?

    _____

    _____

    D. Why might choosing this method be a healthy decision for someone?

    _____

    _____

2. Birth control patch

    A. Effectiveness rate: _____

    B. Estimated cost: _____

    C. How accessible is this method? Is it easy to use?

    _____

    _____

    D. Why might choosing this method be a healthy decision for someone?

    _____

    _____

3. Birth control pill

    A. Effectiveness rate: _____

    B. Estimated cost: _____

    C. How accessible is this method? Is it easy to use?

    _____

    _____

    D. Why might choosing this method be a healthy decision for someone?

    _____

    _____

4. Birth control shot

    A. Effectiveness rate: _____

    B. Estimated cost: _____

C. How accessible is this method? Is it easy to use?

_____

_____

D. Why might choosing this method be a healthy decision for someone?

_____

_____

5. Emergency contraceptive pill

A. Effectiveness rate: _____

B. Estimated cost: _____

C. How accessible is this method? Is it easy to use?

_____

_____

D. Why might choosing this method be a healthy decision for someone?

_____

_____

6. Intrauterine device (IUD)

A. Effectiveness rate: _____

B. Estimated cost: _____

C. How accessible is this method? Is it easy to use?

_____

_____

D. Why might choosing this method be a healthy decision for someone?

_____

_____

7. Vaginal ring

A. Effectiveness rate: _____

B. Estimated cost: _____

C. How accessible is this method? Is it easy to use?

_____

_____

D. Why might choosing this method be a healthy decision for someone?

_____

_____

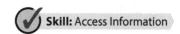

Lesson 24.3   Activity E

Skill: Access Information

Hormonal Methods Research

Instructions: *Find a website or article that provides teen-friendly information about hormonal methods of pregnancy prevention. Answer the following questions to evaluate if this resource is reliable, unbiased, and accurate.*

1. Provide a citation for the website or article you found. Include the website or article name, author, and sponsor.

   _____

   _____

2. Use the following checklist to evaluate the validity and reliability of your research.

   A. _____ Information is current up to one year.

   B. _____ Information is supported by other reliable resources.

   C. _____ Information is based on scientific research.

   D. _____ There is adequate information about the topic.

   E. _____ Facts are cited or referenced.

   F. _____ Information is reasonable (not too good to be true).

   G. _____ Information is applicable to my life stage and situation.

   H. _____ Purpose of resource is stated.

   I. _____ Resource is not making money from the information (not an advertisement).

   J. _____ Author's name is listed.

   K. _____ Author's background is trustworthy and dependable.

   L. _____ Author presents unbiased information.

   M. _____ Resource is sponsored by a credible institution or organization.

   N. _____ Website address of resource ends in .gov, .edu, or .org.

3. After your evaluation, do you think your article is a reliable source of information? Explain.

   _____

   _____

   _____

4. List three facts you learned about hormonal methods of pregnancy prevention.

   _____

   _____

   _____

5. Would you recommend other teens use this website? Why or why not?

   _____

   _____

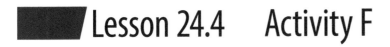 Lesson 24.4   Activity F

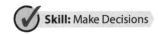 **Skill:** Make Decisions

Choosing Sterilization

Instructions: *Sterilization, a permanent form of contraception, is only appropriate for some adults and can be a difficult decision to reach. Considering the pros and cons of this decision, identify whether sterilization would be an appropriate decision for each of the following scenarios. If you think sterilization is not appropriate, suggest another decision they can make. Explain your reasoning.*

Scenario 1

Manuel and Nikki have been married for about six months. They recently moved to a new city, got new jobs, and started to settle into their new lives. Nikki feels stressed about all of this recent change, and she has been fighting with Manuel more than she used to. Manuel says that they would stop fighting if they had a baby. Nikki wants to have children with Manuel, but is unsure if now is the right time. Nikki suggests sterilization as an option to ensure they do not have any children for whom they are not ready.

1. Would sterilization be an appropriate decision for Manuel and Nikki? Explain your answer.

_____

_____

Scenario 2

Meena recently learned that she has an incurable genetic disease. She does not currently have any children, and has started considering sterilization to ensure she does not pass down her disease to a child.

1. Would sterilization be an appropriate decision for Meena? Explain your answer.

_____

_____

Scenario 3

Before they were married last year, Savannah and James never discussed whether they wanted to have kids. James is starting to feel ready for parenthood, but Savannah has decided she like their life as it is, and does not want children. She thinks James should get a vasectomy and is trying to convince him that he does not want kids either.

1. Would sterilization be an appropriate decision for Savannah and James? Explain your answer.

_____

_____

Scenario 4

Neither Aaron nor Vanessa feels the need to have biological children. Instead, they have chosen to become foster parents. They have temporarily fostered many children over the years, and found more love and satisfaction in that life than they ever expected. Aaron and Vanessa feel their family is complete. Because Vanessa has always experienced severe, negative side effects from hormonal contraception, she is considering tubal ligation.

1. Would sterilization be an appropriate decision for Aaron and Vanessa? Explain your answer.

_____

_____

▰ Chapter 24   Activity G

Practice Test

Completion

Instructions: *Write the term that completes the statement in the space provided.*

1. _____ methods of contraception prevent sperm from traveling through the female reproductive system and fertilizing an egg.

   _____

2. A contraceptive _____ is a device made of plastic foam that contains spermicide and covers the cervix to prevent sperm from entering the uterus.

   _____

3. A small, T-shaped contraceptive device called a(n) _____ device is inserted into the uterus, where it releases hormones that thicken cervical mucus and inhibit ovulation.

   _____

4. _____ contraception can help prevent pregnancy when normal contraception fails.

   _____

5. A(n) _____ awareness method is a contraceptive method that tracks a female's ovulation and avoids sexual activity on days an egg can be fertilized.

   _____

True/False

Instructions: *Indicate whether each statement below is true or false.*

6. _____ *True or false?* Abstinence is the only method of pregnancy prevention that is 100-percent effective.

7. _____ *True or false?* Hormonal methods of contraception protect against pregnancy and STIs.

8. _____ *True or false?* External condoms can be washed out and reused.

9. _____ *True or false?* Getting a diaphragm requires a doctor's examination and prescription.

10. _____ *True or false?* The withdrawal method is an effective form of contraception.

Multiple Choice

Instructions: *Select the letter that corresponds to the correct answer.*

11. _____ Which of the following is a myth about pregnancy prevention?
    A. Latex condoms reduce a person's risk of contracting an STI.
    B. Withdrawal is the least effective method of contraception.
    C. A female cannot become pregnant while menstruating.
    D. Urinating after sex does *not* prevent pregnancy.

12. _____ When using an external condom, _____.
    A. use scissors to open the package
    B. use with petroleum-based lubricant
    C. use a previously-used condom
    D. pinch the condom tip to remove air

13. _____ A(n) _____ can be used for a 30-hour period.
    A. diaphragm
    B. contraceptive sponge
    C. external condom
    D. internal condom

14. _____ The birth control _____ is a thin, two- to three-inch plastic device applied to the skin like a bandage, which releases hormones to stop ovulation.

    A. patch   C. implant
    B. shot   D. pill

15. _____ Which of the following is *not* a fertility awareness method of contraception?

    A. calendar-based methods   C. cervical mucus method
    B. temperature method   D. withdrawal method

Matching

Instructions: *Match each key term to its definition (16–22).*

16. _____ surgical procedure that cuts or blocks the vas deferens, permanently preventing pregnancy

17. _____ contraceptive method that permanently prevents pregnancy by altering the reproductive system, often through surgery

18. _____ substance that inactivates sperm

19. _____ flexible, toothpick-sized contraceptive device inserted under the skin of the upper arm; releases progestin to stop ovulation

20. _____ surgical procedure that cuts or blocks the fallopian tubes, permanently preventing pregnancy

21. _____ cup-shaped contraceptive device made of silicone that covers the cervix to prevent sperm from entering the uterus

22. _____ contraceptive methods that time sexual activity with a female's menstrual cycle and the sexual response cycle to prevent the sperm and egg from meeting

A. birth control implant
B. diaphragm
C. natural methods
D. spermicide
E. sterilization
F. tubal ligation
G. vasectomy

Analyzing Data

Instructions: *The table below portrays data about contraceptive use among high school students from 2019 CDC Youth Risk Behavior Surveillance. Use the information provided to answer the following questions.*

Type of Contraceptive Use	All Students	Male Students	Female Students	Students Who Identify as Heterosexual	Students Who Identify as Gay, Lesbian, or Bisexual
They or their partner used an external condom during last sexual intercourse	54.3%	60.0%	49.6%	56.6%	41.3%
They or their partner used hormonal methods of contraception (including oral contraceptives; an IUD; birth control implant, shot, or patch; or vaginal ring) during last sexual intercourse	30.9%	25.9%	35.2%	31.7%	27.7%
Neither they nor their partner used any contraceptive method during last sexual intercourse	11.9%	10.1%	13.4%	10.1%	25.2%

Centers for Disease Control and Prevention

Figure 1. Contraceptive use among high school students, by sex and sexual orientation

23. Why do you think the rates for external condom use are higher among high school students than rates for hormonal methods?

_____

_____

24. If 20.4 million high school students were sexually active in 2019, how many did not use any method of contraception?

_____

Short Answer

Instructions: *Answer the following questions using what you have learned in this chapter.*

25. What are three factors teens should consider when selecting a contraceptive method?

_____

_____

_____

26. Explain how a vaginal ring works as a method of contraception.

_____

_____

_____